The
15
Minute
Heart Cure

The 15 Minute Heart Cure

The Natural Way to Release Stress
and Heal Your Heart in
Just Minutes a Day

JOHN M. KENNEDY, M.D.,
and JASON JENNINGS

WILEY

John Wiley & Sons, Inc.

Published by John Wiley & Sons, Inc., Hoboken, New Jersey
Published simultaneously in Canada

Design by Forty-five Degree Design LLC

All illustrations appearing in the text are courtesy of Francesca Angelesco.

The information contained in this book is not intended to serve as a replacement for professional medical advice. Any use of the information in this book is at the reader' s discretion. The author and the publisher specifi cally disclaim any and all liability arising directly or indirectly from the use or application of any information contained in this book. A health care professional should be consulted regarding your specifi c situation.

For general information about our other products and services, please contact our Customer Care Department within the United States at (800) 762-2974, outside the United States at (317) 572-3993 or fax (317) 572-4002.

Wiley also publishes its books in a variety of electronic formats. Some content that appears in print may not be available in electronic books. For more information about W iley products, visit our web site at www.wiley.com.

Library of Congress Cataloging-in-Publication Data:

Kennedy, John M., date.

    The 15-minute heart cure : the natural way to release stress and heal your heart in just minutes a day / John M. Kennedy and Jason Jennings.

    p.   cm.
    Includes bibliographical references and index.
    ISBN   978-1-68-162047-3
    1. Heart—Diseases—Prevention—Popular   works. 2. Stress   (Psychology)—Health aspects—Popular works.   I.   Jennings, Jason, 1956– II. T itle. III. Title: Fifteen-minute heart cure.
    RC672.K46 2009
    616.1'205—dc22

                            2009031393

Printed in the United States of America
10   9 8 7 6 5 4 3 2 1

To my wife, Elisa, and two daughters, Emily and Alexa. To my mother, my father, my sisters, and my brother, who taught me to dream big and shoot for the stars.

—Dr. John Kennedy

To Dr. Joel Klompus, our family physician and friend for thirty years.

—Jason Jennings

Contents

Acknowledgments

First, I would like to thank my wife and my two daughters for giving me the time to write this book. Much of the content was inspired by my love for you.

Next, thank you to my parents, my three sisters, and my brother, who have consistently shown me that *anything* we can conceive is possible to achieve.

I have enormous appreciation and gratitude for the many researchers in the field of behavioral cardiology who throughout the years have clearly proven the powerful link between emotional stress and cardiovascular disease. We have come a long way from Dr. Walter Cannon's initial hypothesis that related the hormonal storm of stress to individuals who are "scared to death."

His astute observation that linked the heart and the brain emphasized the powerful negative impact of anxiety and fear on our cardiovascular system. His hypothesis, now established as fact, has contributed greatly to our modern understanding of diseases such as the "broken-heart syndrome" and sudden cardiac death.

I would also like to thank the researchers who recognized early the negative health effects of stress and then took the next bold and necessary next step: showing the powerful healing effects of relaxation therapy.

Thanks to Dr. Herbert Benson, the prolific and renowned Harvard Medical School physician who defined and coined the term *relaxation response*. His career has been committed to the subject, and his unparalleled work ethic and quest to understand stress and how to combat it has led to our modern understanding of this mysterious and complex physiology.

I am especially grateful to those who have consistently supported and endorsed the ancient ritual of relaxation therapy and whose diligent efforts have shaped our modern understanding of health and wellness. Pioneers in the field of integrative medicine, such as Dean Ornish, M.D.; Larry Dossey, M.D.; Andrew Weil, M.D.; Rachel Naomi Remen, M.D.; and Jon Kabat-Zinn, Ph.D., have created a large body of compelling research that proves the merits of managing stress.

Thanks to my patients, who have taught me the importance of recognizing emotional stress as a cardiac risk factor and of teaching patients the B-R-E-A-T-H-E technique as an essential supplement to standard medical care in maintaining superior heart health.

Heartfelt thanks are extended to Sebastian Hitzig, whose courage and strength are a testament to the amazing capacity and awesome power of the mind in healing.

A special thanks goes to Dr. Dean Ornish for his exceptional work in the field of preventive cardiology. His diligent quest has shown that the synergistic combination of Eastern and Western medicine is essential for achieving optimal health.

I am grateful to my special friend and colleague, Dr. Martin Rossman, whose exemplary work in the field of guided imagery has been educational and inspirational. His work has helped countless patients with chronic health conditions like cancer, heart disease, and chronic pain to take a proactive and personal role in the healing process.

Thanks to Francesca Angelesco, an extraordinarily talented and creative artist who has brought life to the concept of *flow* through her healing and soothing artwork.

Thank you to the members of the collaborative and creative team at SmartNow, who are committed to recognizing the relationship of stress and heart disease and who understand the subtleties associated with women and cardiovascular health.

Thanks to our editors, Tom Miller and Christel Winkler, our copyeditor, Judith Antonelli, and our agents, Dan Ambrosio, Kirsten Neuhaus, and Adam Korn of the Vigliano Agency, for their overwhelming support and for understanding the healing power of this book.

Finally, thanks to the teachers, the coaches, and the school administrators who have incorporated the B-R-E-A-T-H-E technique into the curriculum of elementary, middle, and high school students. Heart disease starts early; learning to understand and manage stress will help our youth to enjoy a heart-healthy adulthood. Teaching our children that it is "cool" to recognize what stress is and to learn how to cope with it is a great contribution to their future.

—Dr. John M. Kennedy

My family truly understands the intense nature of my work, and the patience and support they provide see me through the challenging process of writing books.

George Staubli has been the single source of guidance, inspiration, counsel, and encouragement for more than thirty years. Caryn Shehi serves as my personal assistant and organizes my book projects, my schedule, and my speaking engagements. Without her help, I'd be lost. Jeff Marth is my trainer and keeps me healthy. Zamil Sadiq and Ana Baradello challenge me musically and intellectually on a daily basis, and Gene and Judy Nagle take care of Timber Rock Shores, our family lodge on the shores of a secluded lake in the wilderness of Michigan's Upper Peninsula. Mark Powell gets me where I'm supposed to be when I'm supposed to be there, and Bruce Ritter handles financial matters. They're a prized team and wonderful friends.

—Jason Jennings

1

The Heart Cold Facts

It's a proven fact: almost 90 percent of twelve-year-old children in the United States show some signs of atherosclerosis, the disease that causes coronary artery disease, which means you probably have it, too!

Another equally frightening fact is that two-thirds of heart attacks occur in people who have no known history of heart disease. It's an elusive disease with a long lag time and few or no symptoms that, more often than not, strikes without warning. We should all assume that given the way we live and the way we eat, we all have some form of the disease and recognize the importance of protecting ourselves from its unpredictable and harmful course.

In my practice I'm reminded daily of the toxic effects of stress on our hearts. I see countless patients who, immediately after a stressful event, fall prey to the powerful jaws of cardiovascular disease.

The Risk Is Widespread

Examples of stressed-out patients who have been seen in my clinic include an attorney who suffered a massive heart attack on the day of her court trial, a teacher who suddenly developed congestive heart failure after being harassed by disgruntled parents, and a plumber who developed rapid palpitations and a sudden arrhythmia after being accosted unexpectedly by angry clients. In all these scenarios, anxiety from a stressful event caused a sudden flooding of stress hormones that were secreted in high enough concentrations to cause a cardiac event.

Like meteorological weather patterns in a growing tropical storm, life's stresses—whether family, personal, or work-related—can grow, gather momentum, and ultimately wreak havoc on our cardiovascular system. If unrecognized, low-level everyday stress constantly exposes our delicate cardiac tissues to toxic levels of stress hormones, which make our cardiovascular system vulnerable to heart attacks, arrhythmias, and congestive heart failure—the three most common cardiac conditions in the United States.

The most common and studied link between stress and health is with cardiovascular disease. It's estimated that more than 75 percent of visits to primary care physicians are due to stress-related disorders. The mechanisms that relate heart disease to stress are many: increased vascular resistance (higher pressure in the arteries), enhanced platelet activity (thick, clot-prone blood), hypertension (high blood pressure), coronary vasospasm (constriction that limits blood flow), inflammation, electrical instability (erratic heartbeat), and enhanced atherosclerosis (plaque buildup in the arteries). All of these will be discussed in this book.

The Costs in Lives and Dollars

Heart disease and stroke are the most common cardiovascular diseases, and they are the first and third causes of death for both men and women in the United States, accounting for more than 35 percent of all deaths.

More than 870,000 Americans die of heart disease and stroke every year, which is about 2,400 people dying every day. Although these largely preventable conditions are more common among older adults, more than 148,000 (17 percent) of Americans who died of cardiovascular diseases in 2004 were younger than sixty-five. Heart disease and stroke also are among the leading causes of disability in the U.S. workforce. Nearly 1 million people are disabled each year from strokes alone. However, the burden of heart disease and stroke shouldn't be measured only by death and disability.

More than 80 million (one in three) Americans currently live with one or more types of cardiovascular disease or have a serious risk factor that increases the likelihood of developing heart disease. This figure includes 73 million people with high blood pressure, 5.8 million who have suffered a stroke, 5.3 million who have experienced heart failure, 8.1 million who have had a heart attack, and 9.1 million who suffer from regular chest pain (angina pectoris). This year alone, more than 920,000 people will have a heart attack (myocardial infarction), and an additional 780,000 will have a stroke.

More than 6 million hospitalizations occur each year because of cardiovascular diseases. Americans also make more than 81 million doctor visits every year because of cardiovascular diseases. The cost of heart disease and stroke in the United States is projected to be more than $500 billion in 2009, including health care expenditures and lost productivity from death and disability. (In 2008 the cost was $448.5 billion.) As the population ages, the economic impact of cardiovascular diseases on our nation's health care system will become even greater.

The Triggers

As we race through life at breakneck speed, the list of stressful triggers that are linked to cardiac disease is growing. Some of the first reported examples of emotional stressors related to heart disease were depression, anger, and hostility. There's a large body of research from the early 1950s that demonstrates this relationship. More recently, however, because of our fast-paced, multitasking lifestyles, many other emotional triggers have been found to be damaging to the heart. Here are some examples:

Repressing your feelings Marital arguing patterns, for example, have been shown to be detrimental to cardiovascular health, particularly in women. The women who repressed their feelings of resentment and anger toward their husbands had a higher risk of heart attack than those who were more open and expressive of their feelings.

Panicking Panic attacks were also recently found to be linked to the risk of heart attack. In one study, the women who experienced at least one full-blown panic attack had a significantly increased risk of heart attack and stroke.

Experiencing an earthquake The Northridge earthquake that struck Los Angeles in 1994 was one of the strongest ever recorded in North America. There was a sharp increase in the number of deaths from cardiovascular disease immediately after this event, and the researchers postulated that emotional stress from the quake was the cause. Similar data were observed after a major earthquake in Japan.

Worrying while you work Ten thousand British government workers with long-term job stress were followed for twelve years. This study was the first to show that on-the-job stress could cause cardiovascular disease, either directly, from the stress itself, or indirectly, by leading stressed employees to adopt unhealthy lifestyles (such as smoking or heavy drinking). The study found that those with chronic job stress had a 68 percent higher chance of having a heart attack, developing angina, or dying from heart disease.

Having unhappy (or too happy?) holidays   In a twelve-year study conducted in Los Angeles, researchers showed that cardiac death rates were consistently higher in the winter months and peaked at Christmas and New Year's. Specifically, December 25 and January 1 are the deadliest days of the year for heart attacks and sudden cardiac death. The researchers hypothesized that the peak in cardiac deaths during the holidays might be a result of emotional stress, overindulgence, or both.

Being a die-hard sports fan   A study conducted in Germany showed that die-hard soccer fans had an increased risk of heart attack during championship games. When Germany played Argentina during the World Cup games, the researchers observed a threefold to fourfold increase in cardiovascular events for soccer fans. This trend was consistent whether the German team was winning or losing. The stress caused by the suspenseful and exciting games was hard on their hearts.

Feeling terrorized   Researchers in Irvine, California found an increased risk of cardiovascular events in people for three years after the terrorist attack on September 11, 2001. Those who had acute stress responses to the 9/11 attacks had a 53 percent increased incidence of heart problems in the next three years and twice the risk of developing high blood pressure. People who continued to worry after 9/11 had an increased risk of heart problems two to three years after the attack.

Stress Management Improves Both Cardiac Care and Cost

An increasing number of studies, including randomized clinical trials, point to safe and relatively inexpensive interventions that can improve cardiovascular health outcomes and reduce the need for more expensive medical treatments.

A study of patients with heart disease found that psychosocial interventions reduced the risk of further cardiac events by 75 percent, compared to the patients who were given only standard medical care and medications. A sample of 107 patients with heart disease was randomly divided into three groups (standard medical care, exercise, and stress management) and followed for up to five years for the incidence of myocardial infarction, bypass surgery, and angioplasty. The stress management group showed a marked difference compared to the other two groups: only 10 percent experienced these clinical conditions, versus 21 percent in the exercise group and 30 percent in the standard-care group.

An important component of psychological preparation for surgery involves giving patients positive physiological suggestions and imagery. In a randomized, placebo-controlled, double-blind clinical trial, 335 patients were given one of four different audiotapes to listen to before and during surgery. The placebo group listened to a tape with a neutral white noise. Only one experimental tape produced statistically significant benefits; it contained guided imagery, music, and specific suggestions of diminished blood loss and rapid healing. The patients who listened to this tape experienced a 43 percent reduction in blood loss and were able to leave the hospital more than a day earlier than the other groups.

The Chronic Disease Self-Management Program, developed jointly by Stanford University and Kaiser Permanente, includes educational group sessions for patients with chronic disease. The intervention consists of a patient handbook and seven weekly two-hour small-group sessions that focus on developing practical skills to cope with common symptoms and emotions. In a randomized clinical trial of 952 patients, those who participated in the course, compared to the wait-listed control subjects, demonstrated significant improvements at six months in weekly minutes of exercise, self-reported health, health distress, fatigue, and disability. They also had fewer hospitalizations and spent an average of 0.8 fewer nights in the hospital. Assuming that a day in the hospital costs a thousand dollars, the health care savings were approximately $750 per participant—more than ten times the cost of the program.

Not only does stress management appear to reduce the long-term chances that heart patients will have another cardiac event, a new analysis by the Duke University Medical Center and the American Psychological Association demonstrates that this approach also provides an immediate and significant cost savings.

The medical outcomes in this study were notable. Patients in both the exercise group and the standard-care group averaged 1.3 cardiac events—bypass surgery, angioplasty, heart attack, or death—by the fifth year of the follow-up. Those in the stress management group, in contrast, averaged only 0.8 such events during the same period.

The research team found a financial benefit of stress management strategies within the first year of the study. The average cost for the patients who utilized stress management were $1,228 per patient during the first year, compared to $2,352 per patient for those who exercised and $4,523 per patient for those who received standard medical care.

Moreover, the researchers found that the financial benefit of stress management was maintained over time. The average cost rose to only $9,251 per patient during the fifth year for those who used stress management strategies, compared to $15,688 per patient for those who exercised and $14,997 per patient for those who received standard medical care. The average cost per patient per year during the five years was $5,998 for those who used stress management, $8,689 for those who exercised, and $10,338 for those who received standard medical care.

Thus, the benefits of stress management seem to exceed the benefits of both exercise and standard medical care in the reduction of cardiac events *and* in financial costs.

There is now a large body of research that links stress to heart disease, and there is an equally impressive and growing body of evidence of the effectiveness of stress management for successfully treating heart disease. Thus, it seems prudent that clinical interventions should better reflect the emerging evidence of the efficacy and cost-effectiveness of stress management for the treatment of heart disease. Stress management techniques such as B-R-E-A-T-H-E should be an integral part of evidence-based, cost-effective, high-quality health care.

The Data-Treatment Paradox

The substantial evidence of the relationship of stress and heart disease has health care workers, and cardiologists in particular, paying attention. Yet despite this growing body of research, some cardiologists still aren't completely convinced. Why have cardiologists been so reluctant to acknowledge the significance of stress and its relationship to heart health? The role of stress in causing heart disease is still hotly debated in cardiology for two reasons:

1. *Stress is a subjective concept that may be unique to the individual.* What's stressful for one person may not be stressful for another. Some people who are thrill-seekers jump out of airplanes at ten thousand feet and find it pleasurable, whereas others are scared of heights and prefer to keep their feet planted firmly on the ground.

2. *Stress is difficult to measure.* It typically strikes without warning and is difficult to reproduce in a laboratory. After all, how can you measure or control for stress in order to accurately measure its affect on health?

Although most cardiologists believe that stress and heart disease are probably related, they're ambivalent and insecure about discussing the importance of the relationship with their patients. I believe that their ambivalence and lack of acceptance may be due to the following factors:

- A lack of knowledge about supportive data on the relationship between stress and heart disease
- A lack of knowledge about supportive data on the beneficial effects of stress management on cardiac risk
- A lack of motivation to teach stress management due to time constraints
- A perception that stress management methods are ineffective
- A lack of knowledge of how to teach patients specific interventions
- A belief that stress and stress management are not related to their area of expertise
- Poor or no reimbursement for the time spent with patients to explore stress and how it relates to their heart problem.

What cardiologists do agree on is our body's response to stress and the destructive nature of chronic exposure to potentially toxic levels of the stress hormones adrenaline and cortisol.

A Change of Heart

Three recent scientific discoveries that relate stress to heart disease have cardiologists around the world sitting up and taking notice. These measurable, irrefutable, and solid scientific phenomena are as follows:

1. *Neuroimaging* Special neuroimaging techniques, such as magnetic resonance imaging (MRI) and positron-emission tomography (PET) scanning, have allowed us for the first time to visualize the workings of the brain and the heart

under stress. Stress causes a certain part of the brain to become metabolically active, which can be directly imaged using a fancy head scanner known as a PET scan. When subjects with heart disease are given a mental stress test, such as a difficult math problem, their stress hormones become elevated, and the stress portion of the brain lights up on the scan. At the same time, the stress hormones that are released by the anxiety of dealing with the math problem cause the heart to work harder, thus increasing the pulse and the blood pressure and resulting in chest pain or angina. This pattern is reproducible; it confirms the heart-brain connection and illustrates that stress and heart disease are linked.

2. *The broken-heart syndrome*   Another piece of evidence that has caught the attention of cardiologists is the broken-heart syndrome, also known as Takotsubos syndrome. *Takotsubo* is Japanese for "octopus trap." In this syndrome, when the left ventricle of the heart is damaged, the muscle resembles an octopus trap (with its characteristic rounded bottom and narrow neck). For centuries, literary works have been filled with descriptions of characters being stricken by heartache and dying from a broken heart. It turns out that this age-old belief may be scientifically correct.

   The broken-heart syndrome is not restricted to disappointment in love. Extreme grief (such as mourning the death of a loved one) or extreme fear (from being held at gunpoint, being in a car accident, or having to speak in public) are common examples. Even just a stressful argument or a bout of road rage will suffice. In any of these cases, an acute emotional stressor leads to severe, temporary dysfunction of the main pumping chamber of the heart. People who are affected by this peculiar syndrome have surges of stress hormones that cause immediate and measurable destructive changes in the main pumping chamber (the left ventricle). These changes are identical to those caused by a massive heart attack, yet they are reversible.

Those who suffer from this syndrome are usually female and without previous cardiac history. They suddenly experience chest pain and/or shortness of breath after experiencing an acute emotional or physical stress. People with such stress-induced cardiomyopathy have markedly elevated blood levels of adrenaline and noradrenaline.

Although the initial reports of this syndrome were all from Japan, broken-heart syndrome has now been reported in people all over the world. Although the syndrome affects only a small number of people, it clearly shows that a stressful emotional trigger can lead to a flooding by stress hormones and a cardiac event.

3. *Stress as an independent risk factor* A large study at the University of Southern California followed six thousand patients for five years and found that stress and anxiety were better predictors of future cardiovascular events than other traditional risk factors. This is groundbreaking, because it suggests that stress is not simply related to heart disease, it is *independently predictive* of heart disease, just as diabetes or high cholesterol is. This study even showed that patients who were able to reduce their stress level or keep it steady over time were 50 to 60 percent less likely to have a heart attack than the patients whose stress levels increased.

As more and more cardiologists acknowledge the effects of stress on heart disease, an even greater emphasis will be placed on specific stress management techniques like B-R-E-A-T-H-E, which has been specifically designed to decrease cardiac risk.

Is Relaxation Good?

The data clearly suggest that stress is bad for our heart by causing damage from the toxic flooding of the stress hormones adrenaline and cortisol.

If stress is bad for the heart, is relaxation good? The answer, as you might expect, is absolutely yes!

Many of the physiological effects of relaxation are the exact opposite of the stress response. Whereas stress causes your heart rate to rev up and your blood pressure to soar, relaxation causes your heart rate to slow down and your blood pressure to fall. Whereas stress makes you feel anxious, jittery, and sick to your stomach, relaxation makes you feel calm, steady, comfortable, and at peace.

No one can completely avoid stress, but you can counteract it by learning how to evoke the relaxation response, a state of deep restfulness and the polar opposite of the stress response. The relaxation response rests and rejuvenates your body by restoring balance and reducing toxic levels of stress hormones. By consistently activating the relaxation response, the body can begin to repair the damage caused by stress.

Some of the most compelling demonstrations of the positive benefits of relaxation therapy come from Dr. Dean Ornish's five-year study, the Lifestyle Heart Trial (LHT), in which people who made intensive changes in diet, exercise, and stress management had a greater reversal of cardiovascular disease than those who followed a less intense regimen recommended by the American Heart Association (AHA). Those who followed the LHT program had a 37 percent reduction in bad cholesterol, less frequent chest pain, and fewer blockages in the coronary arteries. There were also twice as many cardiac episodes in the AHA program as in the LHT program.

A similar study at Boston's Massachusetts General Hospital, conducted by Dr James Blumenthal, demonstrated that patients with diagnosed heart disease were able to decrease their cardiovascular risk by learning and practicing stress management skills for only sixteen weeks. The patients in the stress management group also had significant increases in heart-rate variability compared to the patients who received standard medical care for coronary heart disease.

Furthermore, after I witnessed thousands of anxious patients about to undergo invasive cardiac procedures, I thought it was important to provide a way for my patients to relax prior to surgery. I therefore designed a study using guided-imagery audio CDs in an attempt to allay patients' preoperative fears. The audio CDs included information about what to expect before, during, and after the procedure and instructions on how to relax by using breathing exercises and visualization. The patients listened to the relaxation CDs before and after the procedure. The results were that the patients who listened to the relaxation CDs felt less anxious, better informed, and generally more satisfied with their care and their doctor. Thus my hunch was correct. When patients felt more relaxed and better informed about their procedure, they reported feeling much less anxious. In addition, the patients who listened to the relaxation CDs had lower blood pressure and a slower heart rate, which may indirectly represent a lower level of stress-hormone release.

Another study showed that patients who were using guided imagery for cardiac surgery had a faster recovery and a decreased length of hospital stay. In 1998, the cardiac surgery team implemented a guided imagery program to compare cardiac surgical outcomes between two groups of patients: with and without guided imagery. Hospital financial data and patient satisfaction data were collected and matched with the two groups of patients. A questionnaire was developed to assess the benefits of the guided imagery program to those who volunteered to participate in it. The patients who completed the guided imagery program had a shorter average length of stay, a decrease in average direct pharmacy costs, and a decrease in average direct pain-medication costs while also maintaining high overall satisfaction with the treatment and the care. Guided imagery is now considered by doctors to be a complementary means of reducing anxiety, pain, and length of stay for cardiac surgery patients.

Summary of Data Supporting the Use of Stress Management and Relaxation Techniques to Decrease Cardiovascular Risk

- Patients who had experienced heart attacks and who were taught relaxation therapies experienced fewer cardiac events in a five-year period. These therapies were taught for only one hour a day for six weeks, and the results were long-lasting.

- An analysis of twenty-seven studies showed that patients with coronary heart disease who were taught relaxation techniques had slower, steady heart rates as well as less angina, fewer arrhythmias, and a lower rate of cardiac events and cardiac death.

- Patients with coronary heart disease who used bio-feedback were shown to increase heart-rate variability, which is a measure of the opposite of the stress response. Biofeedback is a form of relaxation therapy that teaches control of breathing, heartbeat, and blood pressure. Biofeedback is used to combat anxiety disorders and chronic stress.

- Meditation was found to stabilize the heart muscle, making it less irritable and decreasing the number of skipped beats (known as ventricular premature contractions).

- Multiple studies have found that yoga decreases blood pressure in people with high blood pressure.

- Hypnosis was found to stabilize the heart muscle during emotional stress.

- Breath work that involved slow deep breathing was found to lower blood pressure in patients with high blood pressure and to increase heart-rate variability (a measure of the relaxation response) in patients with coronary heart disease.

The data that support the use of relaxation and stress management to decrease cardiovascular risk are growing, but simple techniques are unfortunately few and far between, which is why the B-R-E-A-T-H-E technique is so timely and vitally important.

The Heart: Your Body's Engine

Your heart is a simple pump with four components that work synchronously to maintain the flow of blood to your body's tissues. The four components of the heart are (1) the arteries, the tubes that carry oxygen to the heart muscle; (2) the valves, the doorways that connect the four chambers of the heart; (3) the muscle, the tissue that contracts and propels the blood to the body's tissues; and (4) the electrical system, the internal wiring that creates the rhythm and pulse of the heart.

The heart is like a high-performance engine that requires regular maintenance and servicing. When a part becomes rusty or a spark plug is out, for example, a car is prone to stall, make funny noises, and run poorly. Ignoring the car's need for regular oil changes and general upkeep can lead to periodic breakdowns and eventual engine failure. The heart has similar needs. When part of the heart has a problem, we develop warning signs known as symptoms. Like the engine light in a car, these signs are telling us that our heart needs urgent attention.

A cardiologist, like a good mechanic, analyzes the symptoms, performs the appropriate diagnostics, and troubleshoots to identify the ailing part. The four conditions described below highlight the symptoms that occur when problems arise in each of the four parts. The problems with each of the components correlate with the four most common cardiac conditions.

If the heart had an owner's manual, it would require you to use specific tools to maintain the heart's efficiency. These tools are diet, exercise, and stress management. This book focuses on stress and a specific stress management technique known as cardiac-specific mental imagery. Unlike your neglected car, which can be traded in for a new one when it breaks down, your heart is far less exchangeable. Ignoring the negative effect of stress on your heart poses the risk of irreparable and potentially lethal cardiac damage.

Stress is to the heart what speeding in a residential area is to a car engine: dangerous and hard. Stress management for the heart is like an oil change for a high-performance car. It will serve to keep the heart and the engine running healthy and efficiently.

Two cars of the same make and model are stuck in traffic. One is well maintained, and one is neglected—its service light is on, indicating the need for immediate care. Both cars look shiny and new on the outside. However, looks are deceiving. One car has been serviced and maintained properly to protect the engine from the wear and tear of stop-and-go traffic. The other has been overused and overrun in overdrive with zero maintenance and care, making the engine destined for failure.

Which car is yours?

Like Ice in Their Veins

What do golf champions, Olympic athletes, firefighters, and surgeons have in common? They all display an uncanny ability to focus and execute in the face of adversity, or what most people would consider to be extraordinarily stressful situations.

They seem unaffected by the sheer chaos and mayhem around them. They filter out the extraneous information, the kind that frazzles most humans. They act calmly and coolly, as if they had ice in their veins. How do they do this? Are they genetically superior? Do they possess special gifts? Finding calm in the storm seems almost reflexive to them but is in fact the result of repetition, commitment, and practice. Athletes, surgeons, and firefighters practice regularly so that their seemingly superhuman task is effortless.

This ability, though seemingly extraordinary, is an attribute attainable by all. So, relax, don't worry if you've been accused of being stressed out, neurotic, obsessive-compulsive, or a workaholic. The research in neuroscience has proven that contrary to popular belief, you can indeed teach an old dog a new trick.

Common to all these examples is the commitment to practice, rehearsal, and visualization. Athletes, surgeons, and firefighters imagine the goal, rehearse it in their mind, and then execute it perfectly. When faced with the stressful situation, they call on this muscle memory, which occurs almost reflexively and unconsciously. Athletes describe this state of focus as being "in the zone." Everything around them is in slow motion, which allows them to perform with precision, accuracy, and calm, exactly as rehearsed.

Guided mental imagery is a highly successful and powerful technique that can yield positive results after only a few sessions. My patients have reported feeling a sense of calm and focus after only a single trial. I emphasize to my patients, however, that the greatest benefits can be achieved with practice and commitment. The more dedicated you are to the practice, the more rapidly you will gain mastery of the technique and be able to achieve a sense of calm when you're faced with one of life's unexpected challenges.

More frequent practice will also increase the likelihood of forming cardio-protective emotional memory and ingrained neuron-cardiac nerve networks that will bathe your heart in protective, nurturing, and calming hormones. This ability to find calm in the storm of hormonal stress is what I call opening your heart eyes and becoming heart wise.

How This Book Works

Each chapter in the book details a cardiac condition. Each is illustrated with a story based on real patients (whose names have been changed) and a stressful life event that preceded the onset of their symptoms. Following each example is a cardiologist's analysis, including the diagnosis, the treatment, and the management of the condition. Each chapter concludes with a disease-specific meditation and mental imagery that is metaphorically related to the cardiac condition discussed.

The following are the four most common cardiac conditions:

- *Arrhythmia* This is an abnormal, erratic heart rhythm caused by a diseased electrical system. Arrhythmias can be slow, fast, or erratic. They typically cause symptoms of palpitations, light-headedness, and difficulty in breathing.

  Atrial fibrillation (AF) is the most common disturbance of heart rhythm, and it increases the risk for stroke, heart failure, and all heart-related causes of death, especially in women. AF presently affects more than 2 million Americans and 4.5 million Europeans. The number of patients with AF is expected to increase even more as our elderly population increases.

- *Angina and heart attack* The arteries are three small tubes, no wider than the diameter of a pen or a pencil, that carry precious oxygen from the lungs to the heart itself. In the process we call coronary artery disease, these tubes become progressively narrowed, the muscle is deprived of oxygen, and the person experiences chest pain or angina. When the artery is completely blocked, the blood stops flowing to the heart muscle, and the heart muscle dies in what we call a heart attack.

  According to the Centers for Disease Control in 2006, 24.7 million adults (equivalent to 11.5 percent of the U.S. adult population) have been diagnosed with heart disease.

- *Congestive heart failure* This condition is caused by a severely weakened heart muscle, known as a cardiomyopathy, where the heart becomes unable to contract forcefully enough to deliver blood (and oxygen) to the tissues. In response to the weakened muscle, the blood in the heart becomes congested and, instead of moving forward to the body's tissues, begins to move backward into the lungs, which causes difficulty in breathing. An estimated 5 million Americans currently have congestive heart failure. There are more than four hundred thousand new cases a year, and it's the leading cause of hospital admissions in patients older than sixty-five. The trend has increased threefold in the past decade and is rising.

- *Valvular heart disease*   When the valves, the doors that connect the four chambers of the heart, fail to close properly, they tend to leak or regurgitate. If the hinges become rusty (stenosed, or afflicted with stenosis), the doors don't open properly and pressure backs up like a clogged drain in a sink. The symptoms of valvular heart disease are difficulty in breathing, chest pain, and even passing out.

Aortic stenosis is the most common valve disease. In Scotland, a recent study reported that aortic stenosis is the most common adult heart-valve disease in the Western world. It increases in prevalence with advancing age, afflicting 2 to 3 percent of the population by the age of sixty-five, and its incidence continues to rise.

Your Heart of Gold

Your heart is precious and should be treated with care and regular maintenance. It's arguably your body's most important organ, and a healthy cardiovascular system is essential for enjoying optimal health.

We've made tremendous strides in advancing the technology for cardiovascular care. Devices such as coronary stents, special pacemakers with fancy whistles and bells, and potent pharmaceuticals have all helped to fight heart disease—the number-one killer in America. These therapies are worth every penny, but the cost is still staggering.

Less glamorous yet cost-effective and equally important cardioprotective therapies are exercise, diet, and stress management techniques like the one described in this book. We need to recognize the importance of the latter and make it part of our regular care for the treatment of cardiovascular disease.

Have *a heart of gold*. Learn this simple, cost-effective stress management technique and then teach it to your family members and your friends. Educate them about the powerful negative effects of stress on our cardiovascular system and about the positive, calming, and beneficial cardiovascular effects of B-R-E-A-T-H-E!

By practicing the exercises and techniques herein for fifteen minutes a day, you'll develop the ability to recall the imagery in these exercises when you're faced with an unexpected life stress, and it will protect your heart from the cardio-toxic surge of stress hormones.

2

B-R-E-A-T-H-E

Kara and Tad Kilman both swear that they fell in love and knew they'd be married from the moment that a mutual friend casually introduced them to each other at Cornell University in 1982. Both graduated in 1986 near the top of their class. A big wedding at the top resort in New York's Finger Lakes region soon followed, attended by their delighted families. The couple then headed for Chicago, where new jobs in financial services awaited both of them.

Kara and Tad's plan was to work for ten to fifteen years, pay off their student loans, buy a home, travel, fund their retirement accounts to the max, and then begin a family in their early to mid-thirties.

By 2002, they owned a perfect family home on the North Shore of Chicago, had zero debt, together had saved more than a million dollars in their retirement accounts, and agreed it was time to start the family they had long planned. They decided that Kara would work until she became pregnant and then fulfill her dream of becoming a stay-at-home mom.

The first few years of trying to become pregnant were challenging and filled with more than a few false starts. Each time they failed, Kara and Tad simply smiled, shrugged, and talked about maintaining the "never say quit" attitude that had made them both so successful. However, the faster the biological clock ticked, the more concerned they became about their failure to conceive. The doctors said they were both healthy and there was no reason they couldn't get pregnant. They began reading voraciously on the subject and even tried herbal diets, acupuncture, and reflexology. They were determined to have children.

Eventually they became patients at the Midwest Fertility Center, and after their third attempt at in vitro fertilization (IVF), Kara became pregnant, and the couple was deliriously happy. They spent happy weekends painting and decorating the nursery next to their master bedroom. Their parents, who had been patiently waiting to become grandparents, were overjoyed, and life couldn't have been better.

Their exhilaration ended after their second prenatal visit, when they learned of a placenta problem that would require an early delivery to avoid risk to both Kara and the baby.

Kara immediately took an early maternity leave, and the couple's days were tormented by worry and a seemingly nonstop stream of visits to doctors and ultrasound technicians to monitor the growth and development of their high-risk baby. During a doctor's visit at the five-month mark, the couple's obstetrician raised the possibility of an early delivery, and thoughts of incubators, prolonged hospitalizations, and chronic illnesses began racing through the couple's heads.

In order to determine if the baby's lungs were mature enough for delivery, a small amount of fluid was carefully drawn from

Kara's uterus though a fine tube in a procedure known as amniocentesis. After the procedure, Kara and Tad returned home to await the results. By nightfall, however, Kara had gone into active labor. She was rushed to the University of Chicago Medical Center, where she was brought into an operating room for an emergency Cesarean section, and the baby was delivered.

According to Kara and Tad, the longest and most suspenseful moment in their lives together was waiting for the baby to take his first breath. Finally, after what seemed like an eternity, the baby took a breath and wailed, and a huge sigh of relief and jubilation filled the operating room.

CARDIOLOGIST'S ANALYSIS
Breathing

The story you've just read is fairly common. A fortysomething, highly successful couple desperately wants children, knowing that prenatal risks are higher in older parents. Fortunately, modern medicine allows us to identify and treat potential problems early in the pregnancy, optimizing the well-being of both the mother and the baby. In the eyes of the couple, the first breath of its baby is the most important thing in the world. Arguments, lost sleep, and countless hours spent ruminating and perseverating about the maturity of the baby's lungs have consumed their lives. Finally, the moment arrives, much earlier than expected, and the baby takes the miraculous *first breath*.

The words *first breath* sound cliché, but as every parent will tell you, the first breath is a miracle. It means that the infant's circulatory system is now independent, separate from the mother's. Breathing is essential for life and for bathing our tissues in oxygen. Yet the act of breathing is often overlooked and taken for granted.

Nearly two thousand years ago, a connection between the heart and the brain was recognized by the world's first physician, Galen of Pergamon. The intimate connection between the heart and the brain is essential for understanding stress and how to manage it.

Nevertheless, it's typical for most of us to go through our entire lives taking breathing for granted, never pausing to consider the tremendous significance of the first breath we ever took.

The simple act of breathing is vitally important to my cardiology practice for two reasons:

1. Trouble with breathing is the most common affliction I'm consulted for in my practice. Troubled breathing is caused by heart attacks, congestive heart failure, and abnormal heart rhythms. I have solved the puzzle of troubled breathing thousands of times, but I never grow tired of the priceless reward of helping my patients breathe comfortably again.

2. Learning to acknowledge your breath and to consciously breathe is the *most important* concept in learning to manage stress. Breathing is what allows us to stimulate the relaxation response—the opposite of the stress response.

Becoming conscious and aware of our breathing is one of the fundamental features of the B-R-E-A-T-H-E technique; it reminds us that we have the ability to control our breathing. We can, for example, take a deep breath or a series of shallow breaths, controlling the rate and the depth at will. When we sleep, we become unaware of our breathing pattern. We let the brain take the helm, turn on autopilot, and enjoy a peaceful slumber. If we're lucky, six to eight hours pass without a thought of breathing ever crossing our minds. In order to learn how to relax, we need to become keenly aware of our breathing and realize that both the rate and the depth are in our conscious control.

Hearing the Conversation: The Heart and Brain Connection

When the stress response is triggered, a typical pattern (or reflex) occurs between the heart and the brain. It starts with a trigger: an emotionally charged situation or stimulus.

For example, imagine that you're camping, and upon your return to your campsite you see a large black bear tearing your tent apart. The first thing you'll experience is fear, which activates the amygdala, the emotional center of the brain. The amygdala is sometimes called the primitive brain; it is responsible for emotional responses such as laughing, crying, yelling, screaming, and banging our fists.

The emotional response (the fear) then stimulates the hippocampus, the memory center of the brain. The signal then passes to your midbrain, the hypothalamus, which sets off the true stress fight-or-flight response. This leads to a release of stress hormones, which causes your heart to race, your pupils to dilate, and your blood pressure to soar.

This same pattern and cascade of events occur for less stressful events than meeting a bear, such as being late for work, financial pressures, or having a marital spat. Emotional stress, whether triggered by a frustrating life event or a truly life-threatening one, affects the relationship between the heart and the brain.

The body's heightened response to a life-threatening situation helped us to survive as a species. Our distant ancestors ran from beasts, fought with beasts, and conquered savage enemies; their heroic efforts are why we're here today. However, stress at this level in response to the mundane modern frustrations of paying the bills, sitting impatiently in congested traffic, or weathering the weather delays at the airport can be harmful to your heart.

Stress is bad for the heart. Triggered by fear, stress activates the fight-or-flight response and releases stress hormones that can potentially damage cardiac tissue.

Relaxation is good for the heart. Relaxation is actually *really* good for the heart. The relaxation response, the opposite of the fight-or-flight response, can be elicited by deep, conscious, and focused breathing, which stimulates the vagus nerve (in the cranium), calms and soothes the body, lowers the blood pressure, and protects the heart.

The heart and the brain are in constant communication, and the ways in which our bodies respond to stress (sweaty palms, dry mouth, racing pulse) are a reminder of the conversation between the two organs. This conversation can be likened to a heated argument between two people. When you hear this argument, you should consider it an opportunity to be the peacemaker between the heart and the brain. Use your superb negotiating skills to make order out of chaos by learning the art of *conscious breathing*.

Take a moment to imagine your first breath, and picture what an incredibly beautiful and celebratory event it was. Imagine the reactions of your proud parents and the medical team at your birth. The moment you took your first breath marked the beginning of an important connection between your heart and your brain. What connects these two amazing organs is complex neural circuitry and hormonal control, yet this incredibly elaborate and complicated connection is controlled by the simple act of breathing.

Learning conscious breathing is vital for managing stress and essential for our health and well-being. Galen, the first physician, spoke of the heart and brain as being connected by *pneuma*, or breath. The simple act of breathing is the vehicle that allows us in on this powerful conversation. Stress is bad for the cardiovascular system, and our bodily clues in response to stress are a reminder to us to participate in this conversation and stop stress in its tracks.

Your brain is like the most sophisticated computer on the planet, and it has the B-R-E-A-T-H-E software on its hard drive. Your only challenge is to download the software and activate it. Like all other software, it takes a while to learn, and the more dedicated you are to practice, the more capable you will become at using it to deescalate stressful situations. You should practice breathing daily, with the same kind of training undertaken by an athlete or an artist.

The challenge is to realize when you're stressed and to know that this is your cue to participate in the heart-brain

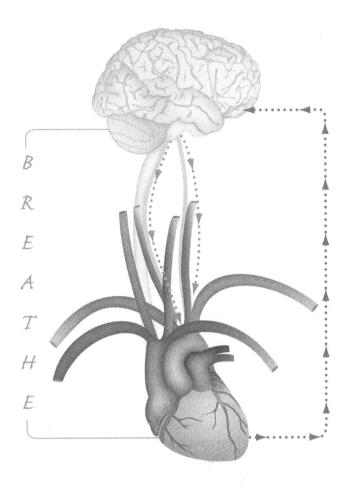

conversation. Instead of responding reflexively with the primitive, emotional brain and becoming worried, anxious, and overwhelmed, you can choose to turn on the B-R-E-A-T-H-E technique.

This conscious choice that can be accessed when you're stressed uses the more advanced brain: the frontal cortex, which allows you to refocus, calm, and soothe yourself in a challenging or even an unexpected situation. Once you recognize that you're stressed, consider it an invitation to "the party"; use the B-R-E-A-T-H-E technique to negotiate between the heart and brain and change the angry and heated conversation into a soothing and calming one.

The B-R-E-A-T-H-E Technique

B-R-E-A-T-H-E is a simple and effective relaxation technique that will help to protect your heart. It is an acronym that stands for Begin, Relax, Envision, Apply, Treat, Heal, End. (These steps are described at the end of the chapter.)

With the coming increase in our elderly population and the fast-paced stressful lifestyle that is typical today, the incidence of heart disease and the cost of health care will continue to rise, and the research has proved a relationship between stress and heart disease. It's time to acknowledge this relationship, recognize stress as an independent risk factor for heart disease, and begin teaching people specific ways to manage stress in order to protect their hearts.

The B-R-E-A-T-H-E technique is the tool that fits the bill; it's easy, effective, and maybe even a little addictive. Some of my patients report that they are "not able to get through the day without it." When you B-R-E-A-T-H-E, feel-good hormones are stimulated, and when you practice regularly, you can lower your blood pressure, decrease your heart rate, and bolster your immune system. When you become stressed and know how to B-R-E-A-T-H-E, you'll develop the ability to quickly and effectively elicit the relaxation response.

The B-R-E-A-T-H-E technique combines two proven relaxation techniques, guided imagery and breath work. Both have been shown to decrease inflammation, decrease the work of the heart (by lowering heart rate and blood pressure), strengthen the immune system, and decrease blood clotting. It's a simple tool that elicits the relaxation response, the opposite of the stress response. To understand how the technique works, let's start with a definition of *breath work* and *guided imagery* and describe how B-R-E-A-T-H-E incorporates both.

Breath Work: Ancient Wisdom Proven by Modern Science

I'm always amazed when I hear that an ancient healing remedy that is derived from plants and has been used for centuries is proven by modern science to have true clinical benefit. Many examples in pharmacology illustrate this point, such as foxglove, which has been used by herbalists since the thirteenth century to treat edema or dropsy, a form of swelling caused by a buildup of fluid. Digitalis, the genus name of foxglove, is also the name of one of the most useful drugs in treating heart disease. It works by making the heart's contractions stronger, and it can also be used to keep the heart from beating too quickly.

Ancient Persian medicine used oil from willow trees for headaches, and aspirin was derived from this centuries later. Opium and cannabis have been used for centuries to relieve pain, long before the scientific tools of today were available to assess their chemical composition and efficacy.

Wisdom and insight about the healing power of breathing is also an ancient and recurring theme throughout the history of medicine, common to many cultures. So too are the potent, toxic effects of fear and worry. The ancient Egyptians, Greeks, Indians, and Chinese all emphasized the premise of this book: that stress is bad and relaxation is good.

It took those of us in the scientific establishment this long to realize that breathing really works. Today, with the advent of MRI and PET scanning, we can finally objectively prove the astute and accurate intuition of our wise ancestors. Heart-rate variability, cortisol levels, and inflammatory markers didn't exist in their days, yet their simple, innate understanding of the power of breathing was absolutely correct.

B-R-E-A-T-H-E uses healing metaphors that emphasize the common theme of *flow*, which is a modern interpretation of several ancient disciplines. *Prana* is a Sanskrit word that means breath, vital energy, and life force. It's similar to the Chinese concept of *chi* (pronounced "chee"), which enters the body with the breath. Prana, like chi, flows through the body, bringing health and vitality, and it is responsible for the beating of the heart and for breathing. Prana is thought to enter the body through the breath and then bathe our tissues through the circulatory system. Prana and chi are both names for the life energy that keeps the body alive and healthy. The concept of breathing, as it relates to circulating healing energy, is known in Greek as *pneuma*, in Polynesian as *mana*, and in Hebrew as *ruach*, which means breath, wind, or spirit.

Deep breathing has a number of healthy physiological benefits: increasing the oxygen intake, the delivery of oxygen to the tissues, and the heart-rate variability while lowering blood pressure and heart rate. Recent studies suggest that deep breathing may also have anti-inflammatory effects.

Guided Imagery

Imagery is the currency of dreams and daydreams; memories and reminiscence; plans, projections, and possibilities.
—Martin L. Rossman, M.D.

The other method used in the B-R-E-A-T-H-E technique is guided imagery, which has also been used for many centuries in health. The Mayans, the ancient Greeks, and the Egyptians all used mental imagery and visualization for maintaining health. Guided imagery, like breath work, can elicit the relaxation response consistently and predictably.

Guided imagery is a proven form of focused relaxation that helps to create harmony between the mind and the body. It helps you to develop calm, peaceful images in your mind and becomes a sort of mental escape. It also provides images that can be stored in your memory and rapidly retrieved in an emergency for use as an effective coping strategy. Many people who are dealing with stress feel a loss of control, fear, panic, anxiety, and helplessness. Research has shown that guided imagery can dramatically counteract these effects.

The Definition of Guided Imagery

Guided imagery is an effective form of relaxation that utilizes the power of the mind to form mental images that can help you to achieve your goals. It is a highly effective therapy that has been used successfully in business, academia, and competitive sports. Top-performing athletes, companies, and scholars all use some form of visualization, or mental rehearsal, to consistently achieve excellence. When guided imagery is practiced regularly, the powerful, beneficial effects that have been achieved for success in business, academia, and sports can also be achieved for health.

In guided imagery, as the name implies, a person is guided with carefully selected words or thoughts through an exercise that is designed to elicit relaxation, stress management, and healing. This form of therapy has been used for health and wellness for centuries and is ingrained in many of the world's cultures and religions. A typical guided imagery session incorporates all the senses: sight, sound, smell, taste, and touch.

Native Americans have used imagery to ward off evil spirits and disease. The ancient Egyptians used imagery in healing rituals, and the Greeks, including Aristotle and Hippocrates, believed that images release spirits in the brain that arouse the heart and other parts of the body.

The most important effect of guided imagery is the promotion of relaxation and the consequent reduction of stress. It's also been shown to improve mood, control high blood pressure, alleviate pain, boost the immune system, and lower cholesterol and blood sugar levels, all of which soothe the heart.

The Types of Guided Imagery

There are a number of different types of guided imagery, but the two that are most relevant to the B-R-E-A-T-H-E technique are relaxation imagery and healing imagery.

Relaxation imagery involves following a script that promotes relaxation. Imagining a calm, soothing, and serene environment, such as a peaceful lake in a quiet woods, can have powerful relaxing effects. Relaxation imagery can counter the stress response and cause measurable declines in blood pressure and heart rate.

Healing imagery is the most relevant to the B-R-E-A-T-H-E technique. It involves imagining the heart as healthy and strong. The exercise uses metaphors that are positive symbols of properly functioning heart parts.

Healing imagery has been used extensively as a complementary therapy for cancer patients. The patients are encouraged to imagine their tumors shrinking, their wounds healing, and themselves as healthy and symptom-free.

Another healing imagery technique is a concept borrowed from traditional Chinese medicine. Chinese medicine believes that illness is the result of a blockage or a slowing of chi, the energy flow in the body, and this blockage makes the body vulnerable to illness and disease. Individuals thus use guided imagery to imagine the energy moving freely throughout the body, as a metaphor for good health.

How Does Guided Imagery Work?

> *Repeated activation of the relaxation response can reverse sustained problems in the body and mend the internal wear and tear brought on by stress.*
> —Dr. Herbert Benson, *Timeless Healing*

The heart and the brain are connected and are in communication at all times. They communicate through the nervous system, the immune system, and the endocrine system. Relaxation is good for the heart because it makes the heart's communications with the brain calm rather than stressful.

Recall that stress causes cardiac damage by releasing hormones that cause the heart to work harder and faster and that stress increases inflammation, which also has damaging cardiac effects.

Relaxation, in contrast, protects our heart through several different mechanisms. The relaxation response is a physiological state of deep rest; it involves both physical and emotional responses to stress that can be elicited by meditation, deep breathing, and prayer.

Herbert Benson, M.D., director emeritus of the Benson-Henry Institute, first described the relaxation response almost thirty-five years ago, and he and his colleagues have pioneered its use in mind-body medicine ever since. Several studies have shown that the relaxation response can help to alleviate hypertension that involves elevated systolic and diastolic pressures.

Elevated blood pressure involves the activation of a special cranial nerve known as the vagus, which means "wanderer." It got its name because it "wanders" all over the body—that is, it communicates through thirteen main branches and connects to four areas of the brain, affecting speech, swallowing, and many other functions—but it is particularly concentrated in the heart and the blood vessels. When the vagus nerve is stimulated by relaxation, the heart rate slows and the blood vessels dilate, resulting in lower blood pressure.

The Benefits of B-R-E-A-T-H-E

In the previous chapter, we cited numerous articles and data to show that stress takes a toll on our cardiovascular system. These are "the heart cold facts."

It logically follows that relaxation has a calming, nurturing, and soothing effect on our heart. Guided imagery and breath work have been used successfully for reducing anxiety, improving coping skills, lowering blood pressure, and decreasing postoperative pain. They have also been shown to have potent immune-bolstering effects. Patients who have used similar techniques have increased their levels of natural killer cells, which are potent immune cells that help to ward off infection. Relaxation therapies such as B-R-E-A-T-H-E lower levels of the stress hormone cortisol, which in large amounts can weaken our body's ability to fight infection and can slow tissue repair.

Here are some heart-warming facts:

- Patients who were taught relaxation therapy after a heart attack had fewer cardiac events in a five-year period than patients who didn't learn relaxation skills.

- A meta-analysis of twenty-seven studies found that patients with known coronary artery disease who were taught relaxation therapy had a slower and steadier heart rate, fewer instances of chest pain, fewer arrhythmias, and fewer cardiac events, including sudden death.

- Biofeedback, a form of relaxation, has been shown to decrease heart rate and blood pressure in patients with known heart disease and to increase heart-rate variability (a measure of the relaxation response).

- Meditation has been proven to decrease blood pressure and abnormal premature heartbeats (ventricular premature contractions).

- Breath work (slow deep breathing) decreases blood pressure and increases heart-rate variability.

- Guided imagery increases heart-rate variability and decreases cortisol (a stress hormone).

- Yoga reduces blood pressure.

In addition to increasing the work of the heart by causing the heart rate and the blood pressure to rise, stress hormones cause two other harmful changes in our body that are linked to cardiac events: inflammation and blood clotting. Relaxation techniques have been shown to decrease both of these and to increase heart-rate variability, which is an objective way to measure the relaxation response.

Inflammation

In the past two decades, research has shown that emotional stress and anxiety are linked to inflammation, and both are linked to heart disease. Hostility and anger have similar links to inflammation and heart disease. Thus, becoming "inflamed"— that is, angry—may have another meaning as well, in terms of your cardiovascular health.

When we become stressed, a special inflammation-causing protein known as IL6 becomes elevated in our bloodstream. The stress hormone adrenaline stimulates the fat cells to release this protein, which leads to the release of cortisol, another potentially inflammatory hormone. Additional substances—such as myeloperoxidase (MPO), an enzyme released by inflamed cells, and C-reactive protein (CRP), another inflammatory marker— are also released into the blood when we become stressed. High levels of both CRP and IL6 were significantly related to an increased risk of coronary heart disease in both men and women. Stress increases inflammation and thus the possibility of a cardiac event.

Thus, stress leads to the release of adrenaline, which leads to inflammation. Inflammation in the blood vessels can cause the rupturing of the artery and the sudden closing of the artery with blood clots. Stress and inflammation have also been implicated in the onset of congestive heart failure and arrhythmias.

Conversely, B-R-E-A-T-H-E's combination of breath work and guided imagery can help to decrease inflammation. When you become hot and inflamed, B-R-E-A-T-H-E will teach you to be calm and cool.

Deep breathing stimulates the vagus nerve. When we inhale deeply, our blood pressure falls very slightly, which is sensed by the brain. The brain then responds to this signal by telling the heart to increase its rate. When we exhale, the opposite occurs: our blood pressure rises slightly, which is sensed by the brain and leads to a decrease in heart rate. Deep breathing causes a cyclical pattern of variation in our heart rate: up when we inhale and down when we exhale. High heart-rate variability is a sign of vagus nerve activity, which is the opposite of the stress response. Low heart-rate variability is associated with higher cardiovascular mortality. Slow, deep breathing increases heart-rate variability and vagus nerve activity—the opposite of stress.

Another way that relaxation protects our heart is through our immune system. Current research shows that stress activates inflammation, which has been implicated as a cause of heart disease. Relaxation has been shown to decrease inflammation, and current research suggests that the vagus nerve may be the link that protects our heart.

Data from the Netherlands describe a two-way freeway, of sorts, that connects the heart and the brain. This model proposes that signals known as cytokines are released from the heart as warnings of inflammation. These signals are transmitted to the brain on the "northbound" portion of the vagal freeway. The brain receives the warning signals and sends a rescue message back, down the "southbound" vagal freeway, which blocks the inflammation process and thus decreases atherosclerosis (plaque buildup in the arteries).

Deep breathing, when practiced correctly, elicits the relaxation response, the opposite of the fight-or-flight response, by increasing heart-rate variability and possibly blocking inflammation.

Other Proven Benefits of the B-R-E-A-T-H-E Technique

We know that chronic untreated stress weakens our immune system and increases inflammation and our risk for cardiovascular disease. We also know that depression, anger, and anxiety take its toll on our hearts; this can cause thickened blood, which is prone to clot. The platelets, which are responsible for blood clotting, become sticky, which is one explanation for the increased cardiovascular risk in depressed patients.

In December 2006, ABC News reported a study from the *British Medical Journal* that activities that promote slow and deep breathing can positively alter many of the body's vital signs. The same year, an American Heart Association study reported that simple workplace interventions can reduce the impact of stress on the heart. Office workers were able to achieve significant changes in heart-rate variability and a small decrease in arterial blood pressure by participating in stress management.

As a way of dealing with stress, American workers often engage in unhealthy behaviors, such as excessive comfort eating and other poor dietary choices, smoking, and physical inactivity. The global workforce is becoming overweight, sicker, and less productive due to chronic conditions such as heart disease and diabetes. B-R-E-A-T-H-E is the perfect tool at the perfect time for the American workforce: it's a simple way to combine guided imagery and relaxation therapy with meditation and breathing work. Take a look at some of the proven benefits.

Benefits of Guided Imagery and Relaxation Therapy

- Lowers blood pressure
- Bolsters the immune system
- Increases parasympathetic tone (the opposite of the stress response)
- Improves concentration and focus
- Decreases anxiety and pain
- Decreases the production of cortisol (a stress hormone)
- Decreases the required dosage of pain medication for postoperative heart surgery patients

Benefits of Mindful Meditation and Breath Work

- Increases heart-rate variability
- Increases the production of endorphins and enkephalins (natural painkillers)
- Decreases the production of cortisol
- Improves concentration and focus
- Decreases the production of adrenaline (a stress hormone)

Positive Thinking as Preparation
for B-R-E-A-T-H-E

In order to achieve optimal results, a preexercise routine, or a sort of mental preparation, is recommended. In football this is a pregame pep talk; in golf, the preshot routine; and in business, it's the CEO's talk to the company employees. All are planned preparatory routines that will achieve the best results.

A golf metaphor best describes getting ready to B-R-E-A-T-H-E. In golf, the swing coach provides the golfer with helpful reminders or ideas, known as *swing thoughts*, that help one to play well throughout the eighteen holes. Think of life as a challenging championship golf course filled with potential trouble at every hole: sand traps, waste bunkers, and water hazards abound. To navigate successfully through the daunting course of life, your "swing thought" must be to stay positive, relax, and let everything flow.

It's a simple concept, but it's actually quite profound. Staying positive is very advantageous to your health. Emotional vitality is a positive state associated with interest, enthusiasm, excitement, and energetic living, and this attitude has been shown to protect people from heart disease. A study from the Netherlands found that people who are pessimistic are more likely to die of heart disease. Moreover, people who are optimistic feel better and live longer than people who aren't. It has been speculated that optimists are relatively immune to heart disease because they cope with stress better. They quickly defuse the stressful situation by using techniques like B-R-E-A-T-H-E, which in the long run protect their hearts.

Reading each chapter of this book will not only help you to understand the workings of your heart, it will also introduce you to compelling familiar stories that will convince you that you're not alone. Make an effort to involve your family or support group in this process. Studies show that people with lonely hearts or poor social networks have an increased risk of developing heart disease. Teach your family, friends, and loved ones about this technique. Share the stories and exercises with them, and you'll be one big heart-healthy family.

Learning the signs, symptoms, diagnoses, and treatments of the various cardiovascular diseases will empower you and help you to understand the negative impact of stress on your heart and, more important, the powerful healing and soothing properties of the B-R-E-A-T-H-E technique.

In my practice I've found that the patients with the most successful and vigorous cardiovascular health are those who seek a thorough understanding of their disease and remain positive, informed, and committed to the therapeutic plan. Such patients have consistently superior therapeutic results, compared to those who are uninvolved and apathetic about their disease.

Even if you're a naysayer and have a negative view of the world, learning to be positive is still possible. Research on learning and memory has shown that even the most rigid, stubborn, and stifled individuals are capable of learning to be positive. Our brains are much more malleable than we once thought.

A recent study has proved the importance of emotional vitality in maintaining optimal cardiovascular health. It followed six thousand men and women for fifteen years; during this time, twelve hundred developed coronary heart disease. Even after allowing for traditional cardiac risk factors, the study demonstrated that patients with positive attitudes and higher emotional vitality were less likely to develop heart disease. The researchers speculated that the patients with a more positive attitude and higher emotional vitality had better coping mechanisms for dealing with unexpected life stress.

It's easy to say, "Just have a positive attitude," but a positive attitude depends on several factors, like genetics, social support, and health habits. Some of these are not changeable, but we now know that even the most negative and pessimistic people can learn ways of thinking to maintain a positive mindset, and a positive mindset bolsters your immune system.

No matter what a person's age or sex, the human brain is much more malleable than we once thought. Thus, when you practice the B-R-E-A-T-H-E technique, remember to begin your exercise with positive thoughts. It feels good, bolsters your immune system, and strengthens your heart.

Here are some additional things you'll need before you begin:

- Comfortable, loose-fitting clothing
- A quiet place where you will be uninterrupted for fifteen minute

The Elements of B-R-E-A-T-H-E

As we noted earlier, B-R-E-A-T-H-E is an acronym. Each of the letters represents one of the seven steps that make up the technique. For best results, follow the simple template below. Remember that conscious breathing is what connects the heart and the brain and allows us into the conversation between the two organs.

B: Begin

Every book, song, poem, and exercise has a beginning. Begin your exercise daily in the most ideal place at the most ideal time for your schedule. For example, a truck driver can do this while sitting quietly on the loading dock just before checking the inventory and planning the daily delivery route. A surgeon might do it while scrubbing for surgery. If you work in an office setting, try taking a short walk at lunch to a quiet place, away from the frenzied workplace, to practice.

You might choose a quiet place in your home and practice soon after waking, which can help you to focus and achieve your daily goals. Some people use the B-R-E-A-T-H-E technique just before climbing into bed, which helps them to relieve racing thoughts and to achieve more quality sleep. Wherever and whenever you decide to B-R-E-A-T-H-E, be sure to practice the same way each time. Try to develop a rhythm and a routine in your practice.

When you begin, pick a quiet and cozy place, where you won't be interrupted for fifteen minutes, which is the amount of time you need to gain mastery and optimize the results of the B-R-E-A-T-H-E technique. Begin your exercise with a positive attitude, knowing that this fifteen minutes is a well-deserved gift to yourself.

R: Relax

This might seem counterintuitive, but relaxation actually requires concentration and focus. It's not like sinking into a beanbag chair, flipping on the TV, and ripping open a bag of chips. To elicit the relaxation response requires focused and conscious breathing. Try to clear all thoughts when you start, and concentrate only on your breath. Recall that focused, controlled, and conscious breathing is what allows us into the conversation between the heart and the brain. A helpful tool is to imagine a beautiful hiking path that is very familiar to you; with each step you take, you become more and more relaxed. The end of this familiar path is always the same peaceful and serene place at the foot of a majestic flowing river.

Conscious Breathing

1. Sit in a comfortable chair with arm rests, and let the gravity of your body sink right into it. Your body should be as relaxed as possible. Feel the weight of your arms and legs supported by the chair. Feel your feet comfortably in contact with the ground.

2. Pay attention to your breathing. To help focus on your breathing, place one hand on part of your chest or abdomen and watch your hand rise and fall with each breath.

3. Inhale through your nose, if possible. If not, breathing in through your mouth will suffice.

4. Inhale deeply and slowly (through your nose) and feel it in your abdomen. You'll see and feel your abdomen rise with each inhalation. Your chest should move only slightly.

5. Exhale through your mouth, keeping your lips, tongue, and jaw relaxed. Extend your exhalation, if you can, to a count of seven—like the number of letters in the word B-R-E-A-T-H-E.

6. Relax and focus on the sound and feeling of long, slow, deep breaths.

7. Listen to the conversation between your heart and your brain. As you inhale, notice your pulse slightly increasing; as you exhale, your heart rate will decrease.

Repeat a series of seven breaths, and you will notice that you feel deeply relaxed. You'll know it's time to go on to the next step in B-R-E-A-T-H-E when you feel all your muscles relaxed and your entire weight supported by your chair. The more you practice, the easier conscious breathing becomes. After a few practices, this technique will become routine, and you can spend more of your energy focusing on the second component of the B-R-E-A-T-H-E technique: the heart-healing guided imagery.

E: Envision

Visualizing an end or a desired goal is common practice in sports, business, and academics. The most innovative and successful companies today rely heavily on dreaming, imagining, and thinking "outside the box." Without imagination we would never progress. Wireless technology, the Internet, and all scientific breakthroughs are born out of an active imagination. As in business and in sports, imagination has important applications in maintaining health and wellness.

When you practice your B-R-E-A-T-H-E exercises, imagine your heart parts as healthy and strong. Imagine all four parts: the arteries, the muscle, the valves, and the electrical system.

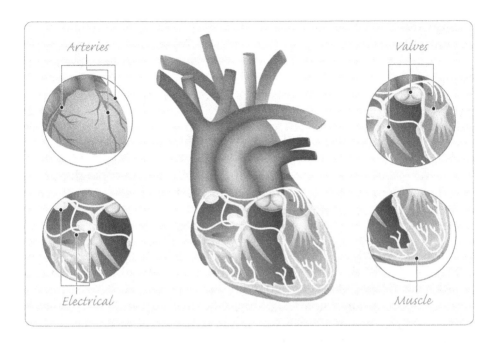

Arteries

Valves

Electrical

Muscle

Analyze what they look like and how they work together in unison to provide the constant, unimpeded flow of blood to nourish your entire body. Studies show that patients who have a thorough understanding of their medical condition and use visualization have better overall health.

Once you've learned the healing metaphors in the heart exercises in this book, envision how they soothe and calm your body and allow your heart to rest and idle. Visualize your heart as strong and powerful, with all the parts working synergistically and efficiently. Remember that guided imagery exercises lower your heart rate, lower your blood pressure, reduce cortisol output, and strengthen your immune system.

A: Apply

When you read through the guided imagery exercises in the following chapters and observe the accompanying art, imagine how the heart-healing images and metaphors can be applied to and related to your healthy heart. Stay focused, concentrating on the significance of the images, because it is easy to become distracted.

If you lose focus, you will probably feel a little anxious or frustrated. Don't worry, because it's easy to get right back on track. The bodily feelings that stress creates are the reminder of the heart-brain conversation and an invitation to stop stress in its tracks. Apply the principles of the technique and recall that conscious breathing is the way back into the conversation. This should help you to refocus.

The apply step in B-R-E-A-T-H-E has two facets. The first is to apply the meaning of the metaphors to an efficiently working heart. The second is to apply this technique in times of heavy stress and use it as an effective coping mechanism. If you practice regularly, each heart-healing metaphor will be filed away in your memory bank. These memories will be accessible, retrievable, and very helpful in breaking the cycle of stress.

T: Treat

The B-R-E-A-T-H-E technique is a pleasurable and therapeutic exercise. You deserve this enjoyment and gratification. These fifteen minutes will make you feel revitalized and energized. This exercise is not like a chore, a duty, or an errand to check off your to-do list. It is an extremely pleasant and comforting experience that you will begin to look forward to. Practicing regularly is like exercising in the gym; it will foster feelings of elation, happiness, and feelings of bliss—but with much less physical effort! The B-R-E-A-T-H-E technique is more like a spa treatment than a physical workout. Your entire body will feel deeply relaxed and invigorated.

H: Heal

The B-R-E-A-T-H-E technique is healing. By practicing fifteen minutes daily, you will train the neural networks that connect your heart and your brain. You will consistently elicit the relaxation response, which has a number of healing physiological responses, including increased heart-rate variability, decreased blood pressure, enhanced immune response, and lower pulse rate. B-R-E-A-T-H-E can be used anytime and virtually anywhere. It is accessible to anyone and simple to learn. Relaxation therapy has been shown to decrease arrhythmias, improve focus, improve sleep, and improve our blood sugar and cholesterol levels. Recalling the healing properties of this pleasurable exercise will help you to remain positive and focused.

E: End

Every effective exercise has a formal beginning and ending. When you have successfully completed your exercise and carefully and mindfully focused on all of the heart-healing metaphors, you will feel deeply relaxed. You will also feel energized, revitalized, and ready to face the rest of the day. This is because you have actively concentrated on the rhythm and the rate of your breathing, which increases the spread of oxygen to your tissues. You have also concentrated on the improved flow of oxygenated blood to your tissues and on an efficiently working healthy heart.

Before you end, make a mental checklist of the healing metaphors you studied in your exercise and begin to notice your surroundings. Imagine how you might use this work throughout your day to help defuse a difficult situation. Think of how the ending of your exercise is really the beginning of your day and how this cycle is like the cycles of your breathing and your heart function.

Remember that the combined guided imagery and breathwork exercises in each chapter were carefully crafted and are filled with heart-healing metaphors that relate to the properly functioning heart parts. Similar to the concept of chi in Chinese medicine, the B-R-E-A-T-H-E exercises emphasize how flow relates to an efficient, healthy, and smoothly running cardiovascular system. B-R-E-A-T-H-E helps to unblock the heart parts and promotes flow in the electrical, valvular, muscular, and arterial systems. In order to reap all of the many health benefits of the B-R-E-A-T-H-E technique concentrate on staying positive, being relax, and flowing with everything.

Follow-up

A very healthy Jeremiah Kilman, also known as "the terror of Hull Terrace" and the son of Kara and Tad, started preschool at the North Shore School in September 2009. Devorah, his baby sister, was born in 2007. Their parents faithfully practice the B-R-E-A-T-H-E technique daily and credit the reduced stress in their life for their easy second pregnancy.

3

Treating and Preventing Congestive Heart Failure

Amy Meyers knew that her life was about to change for the better as she smiled and boarded United Airlines flight 21 at JFK Airport to fly from New York to Los Angeles. For two years she'd been quietly wooing one of Hollywood's hottest talents to do a syndicated daytime talk show for the network, and it looked as if he was finally going to agree to do the show. "Move over, Ellen, Maury, and Jerry," she thought to herself as she sank into the luxurious first-class seat on the morning flight, "and watch your backside, Oprah, because this is going to be the biggest daytime television blockbuster of all time, and I'm the one who's going to pull it off." She'd never been more nervous, excited, and anxious in her life.

Amy's six-thirty flight was set to touch down in Los Angeles at nine-thirty. With no bags to retrieve and a car waiting for her, she would easily make the eleven o'clock meeting at the agent's Wilshire Boulevard offices, and with any luck the deal would be done by noon and the press releases would start flying.

"Welcome aboard," said the young male flight attendant. "May I get you some orange juice, champagne, a mimosa, or something else to drink?"

It was too early for a drink, but since Amy was facing six long hours in flight and hoping to sleep for most of them, she reasoned that liquor would help her sleep, so she asked for a Screwdriver (vodka and orange juice). The first drink made her a little woozy, so when the flight attendant asked if she'd like another, Amy decided that one more would definitely help her to sleep. She sipped the second drink, while slowly nibbling from the dish of salted peanuts that the flight attendant kept refilling, and declined breakfast. Before she knew it, she was nodding off to sleep, somewhere between thinking and dreaming about the surprising turns her life had taken.

Amy had been the first person in her family to go to college. Nobody—her parents, her older brothers and sisters, her aunts and uncles and cousins—had ever moved farther than twenty-five miles away from tiny Worden, Illinois. Her father, a rural postal carrier, always laughingly described his high-strung daughter as being "as stubborn as a donkey and smart as a whip," and her stellar academic performance in the local unified high school district paid off with a full academic scholarship to Northwestern University. By juggling scholarships, student loans, three part-time jobs, and the lack of financial help from home, she graduated in 1990 with a stellar grade-point average and an armful of letters of introduction and recommendations from her professors and former employers attesting to her determination.

Amy headed to New York and swiftly landed her first job as an assistant editor at a publishing company, where she corrected manuscripts in return for an anemic salary that required her to share a shabby two-bedroom apartment with three roommates.

She didn't mind, however. New York was everything she'd ever dreamed it would be, and she and her midwestern roommates thrived on each new discovery and accomplishment, constantly laughing and promising one another that one day they'd all be important and running the show.

Her first job quickly led to an editor's position, followed by a stint at a dot-com that failed, shaking her badly; a position in charge of new media for a small advertising agency; and a job in which she helped to produce and manage a new Web site that aired serial comedic vignettes.

Amy's world changed when NBC's *Today Show* aired one of the video spoofs she'd produced, and she was asked to join CNN as the producer of a planned copycat version of *The Daily Show*. The program never got off the ground, but Amy leveraged the position into other television jobs, and eventually, by age forty, she was indeed running the show and in charge of television syndication for Fox Television.

Along the way there'd been more than a few men, but no keepers. Most men weren't able to handle her drive and ambition, and those who weren't intimidated *by* her were intimidating *to* her.

In a city where everyone seems to have a gym membership and lug a giant water bottle around, Amy was the exception. She had started dozens of exercise regimens, but there never seemed to be enough time to stick to any of them. She counted on her nervous energy, lots of caffeine, and not much food to keep her weight in check, which had allowed her to remain a minuscule size 4. Twelve-hour work days followed by evening business meals, at which she'd indulge herself with a few glasses of wine and limit her food intake by picking at the protein in the entrée, were the norm. Food and exercise didn't matter to Amy. She didn't have time.

Long before she expected it, she felt a gentle hand on her shoulder. "It's time to wake up, Ms. Meyers. We're going to be landing in a few minutes."

Amy sat up in a momentary panic, wondering where she was and what was happening. Her heart seemed to give a quick lurch as she moved her seat forward into an upright position and tried to shake off the sleep. Deciding that some cool water on her face and some makeup would revive her; she bent forward to pull on her shoes and discovered she couldn't get them on her feet. Her feet had swollen on long flights before, but never like this. "The heck with it," she thought. "I'll go to the bathroom first and then figure out how to fit my feet into the shoes." She padded to the front of the cabin in her bare feet.

As she stood before the bathroom mirror, rinsing her face and putting on a touch of makeup, the immensity of the coup she was about to pull off hit her, and she felt a sudden wave of anxiety sweep through her body like a lightning bolt.

"Damn, my feet are swollen like an old lady's feet," she whispered to herself, as she struggled to get her shoes on. Only after a fierce struggle did she finally manage to get them on, and as she surveyed the swollen folds of flesh above the edges of her shoes, she knew that walking was going to be a real effort.

When the doors of the plane opened, Amy stood up, clumsily grabbed her overnight bag from the luggage bin above, and headed toward the door, doing a pigeon walk in shoes that were killing her. By the time she made it to the end of the Jetway, she realized that she was short of breath and her heart was racing, as if it were going to jump out of her chest.

Once she stepped into the terminal, she stopped, put her bag down, and instinctively leaned forward and placed her hands on her thighs to try and gain control of the situation. The first thought that occurred to her was that she was having a panic attack like the one she'd had in college before a stressful final exam. "No way am I going to let a stupid panic attack screw this meeting up," she thought to herself. She took a few deep breaths, felt a little relief, stood up, and made her way to where a car was waiting for her.

Walking was horrible. Her swollen feet didn't want to cooperate, and she felt weak-kneed, but at least her pounding heart seemed to have returned to a normal rhythm. Breathing was still a struggle. She couldn't seem to inhale a deep breath, only short shallow breaths. As she walked through the baggage claim area, she saw a driver holding a sign with her name on it, so she hobbled up to him, gave him her bag, and without even uttering a "good morning," she said, "Let's get going. Where's the car? I can't be late for my meeting."

The driver smiled and said, "Good morning, Ms. Meyers," dismissed her as another self-important and entitled New Yorker, and added, "I'll get the car, if you want to wait here for just a few minutes." Feeling increasingly irritable, she snapped, "Hurry up, I don't want to be late."

Most arriving passengers who are lucky enough to be picked up by a car service at the Los Angeles airport will walk with the driver to the car and be out of the airport in a few minutes. However, when the driver has to retrieve the vehicle and drive around the airport to pick up a passenger, the minutes can begin mounting, as they did that morning.

By the time the driver returned to the United Airlines terminal, nearly thirty minutes had passed. During this time, Amy had started panicking about two things: Would she be late for the most important meeting in her life? Was there something seriously wrong with her?

As she walked the few feet to the car, she looked down and saw that her ankles were even larger than they had been on the plane, and her heart had started a foreboding, rapid pounding again that made her want to jump out of her skin and run. She wanted to get in the car, sit back, close her eyes, relax, and have everything become normal again. She wanted this more than she'd ever wanted anything in her life.

The cool, relaxing oasis that Amy hoped to find inside the car wasn't there. She couldn't sit still; she was growing increasingly angry with the driver for no reason, and she didn't know why. She kept forcing herself to close her eyes and silently repeat, "I am okay, this will go away. I am okay, this will go away. I am okay, this will go away." It didn't.

"Are you all right, Ms. Meyers?" asked the driver.

"I'm fine," she fired back. "Just get me to my damn meeting, will you?"

As the driver exited the airport and pulled onto the highway, both the driver and Amy looked ahead and saw the same thing at the same time. The freeway was a parking lot; not a single car was moving.

"You are goddamned incompetent for bringing me this way," she accused the driver, knowing that she was going to be late for her meeting. "I don't care how you do it, but get us off this freeway and get me to my meeting."

The driver looked in the rearview mirror before he started to explain that there was no way off until the next exit, and what he saw shocked him. Amy Meyers was foaming a pink froth out of her mouth, and she had the look of a wild woman with bulging, terror-filled eyes.

"Dispatch, this is Carl in limo 46," screamed the driver into his radio. "I'm stuck on [Interstate] 405 at Century Boulevard, and I need an ambulance immediately for my passenger. Call 911 fast!"

Sheer terror had overtaken both Amy and the driver. As he pulled off the highway onto the shoulder, she was screaming that she couldn't miss her meeting, her mouth was foaming voluminous amounts of froth, and her lips were turning blue. The driver jumped out of the car and opened the back door to try to help, but didn't know what to do. Within less than a minute he heard a siren in the distance and prayed it was headed their way. Drivers in other cars slowly rolled by with their windows down and were shouting offers of help.

Amy lay on the back seat, her clothing disheveled and her body almost convulsing as she fought to breathe. She felt as if she were drowning. The siren grew louder, and the driver saw an ambulance making its way toward them down the shoulder of the road a quarter mile away. Before the driver knew what was happening, he was being shoved aside by two burly paramedics, who were lifting Amy out of the backseat and onto a gurney. Rubberneckers had stopped traffic completely.

The paramedics suspected that they were dealing with florid pulmonary edema, and her pulse was rapid and irregular strongly suggesting a potentially lethal heart arrythmia (abnormal heart rhythm). The paramedics quickly put an endotracheal tube down Amy's throat for a portable ventilator, and another paramedic stood by, ready to begin administering lifesaving drugs the moment the word came from the cardiologist on the emergency room radio. California Highway Patrol officers had finally arrived and were frantically trying to clear a path so the ambulance could get off the freeway and onto a surface road.

At first Amy tried to fight off the paramedics, but she finally gave up. Then, in what appeared to be a valiant effort to regain her composure, Amy heaved herself up against the straps that were holding her to the stretcher and fell back. Her head rolled to the side, and to everyone watching, it appeared that Amy had died.

The paramedics and police officers redoubled their efforts, loading her into the ambulance with shocking speed, and as the sirens screamed, the team began heroic efforts to shock Amy's heart back into rhythm. They were seven minutes from the hospital, where another team stood ready to receive the patient. Despite everyone's best efforts, Amy didn't regain consciousness, and all efforts to resuscitate her failed. She was pronounced dead shortly after arriving at the UCLA Medical Center.

Amy Meyers was forty years old. One week later, during funeral services at Trinity Lutheran Church in Worden, Illinois, the church's pastor called Amy's passing a tragedy. We agree.

CARDIOLOGIST'S ANALYSIS
Congested on the Highway

Congestive heart failure occurs when the heart muscle weakens and it is unable to generate enough force to propel blood forward to the brain and the body. Instead, the blood backs up and flows backward into the lungs. The heart, like our patient stuck in traffic on I-405, becomes congested.

When the heart muscle is working normally, it contracts forcefully and propels blood to the brain and throughout the body with each beat. When the muscle is weakened, the heart loses its ability to contract, causing blood to back up in our lungs, abdomen, legs, and feet. The heart becomes so weak that it's unable to generate the force required to pump the blood to the brain and the body; as the blood backs up into the lungs instead, it causes a feeling of suffocation.

The patient is stuck in standstill traffic, so to speak, unable to get to her important meeting on time. As her anxiety increases, so do her blood pressure and heart rate, which causes her heart to become congested. As her blood pressure rises and her heart races, the blood becomes more and more backed up, which causes fluid buildup in the lungs and blocks oxygen from entering the bloodstream. She becomes more and more anxious, and begins to gasp for breath and feel as if she were drowning.

An estimated 5 million Americans currently have congestive heart failure. There are more than four hundred thousand new cases a year, and it's the leading cause of hospital admissions in patients older than sixty-five. The trend has increased threefold in the past decade and continues to rise. The average annual cost to treat congestive heart failure is more than $32 billion.

Patients who are prone to this condition have a damaged heart muscle and are given the diagnosis of cardiomyopathy. *Cardio* means "heart," *myo* means "muscle," and *opathy* means "disease": cardiomyopathy, the disease of the heart muscle.

The causes of a weakened heart muscle, or cardiomyopathy, are poorly controlled high blood pressure, viruses, blocked coronary arteries, leaky and blocked heart valves, excessive alcohol, and low thyroid hormone levels.

Failing Pump: Signs and Symptoms

Common symptoms of congestive heart failure include fatigue, shortness of breath, racing and erratic heartbeats, and swelling of the feet, the abdomen, and even the face. Other common symptoms of congestive heart failure are as follows:

- Weakness, tiredness
- Difficulty breathing when you are lying down
- Waking up at night coughing or with difficulty breathing
- Needing to use the bathroom many times at night
- Dizziness

Lethal Cocktail: Salt, Alcohol, and Stress

Patients with a history of congestive heart failure have a weakened heart muscle, which is vulnerable to excess fluid and has difficulty maintaining the body's delicate fluid balance. Our patient committed the ultimate sin of consuming salted nuts washed down with two drinks in order to soothe her anxiety. Her heart muscle became like an overstretched balloon that lost its elasticity and its ability to recoil and contract. This made it vulnerable to fluid overload. Salt consumption causes further fluid retention, which becomes too much for the weakened heart to handle; this in turn leads to the swelling of the ankles, the abdomen, and the feet. When fluid builds up in the lungs, the oxygen in the blood becomes compromised and the patient becomes short of breath. In severe cases the patient begins to cough up pinkish, frothy sputum, known as pulmonary edema, or water on the lungs.

Like salt, alcohol is harmful to the heart, but in two different ways. First, it tends to dehydrate the body, making you feel thirsty. Consuming more fluid into an already filled container increases the risk for congestion and fluid overload. Second, alcohol can lead to hypertension, which places a further stress and load on the heart. Alcohol is a direct toxin to the heart muscle, further weakenening its ability to contract.

This scenario represents a classic example of a patient with a weakened pump who ingested a potentially lethal combination of salt and alcohol. When these conditions are combined with a stressful life event, the patient develops congestive heart failure, requiring emergency medical attention.

Congested Heart and the Vicious Cycle

When the heart is damaged by prolonged high blood pressure, alcohol, or a virus, it pumps with less force, and less blood moves through the body. In an attempt to compensate for the weakened pump and to maintain the same amount of blood moving through the body, a number of physiological changes occur. Hormones, such as adrenaline, aldosterone, and angiotensin, are released in order to maintain blood pressure and flow. These powerful chemicals cause the blood vessels to constrict and salt and water to be absorbed.

Unfortunately, when these chemicals are released, they only make matters worse. When the pump begins to fail, less blood reaches the kidneys, so the kidneys respond by releasing a hormone that is responsible for retaining water and salt. This extra fluid is frequently too much for the failing heart and causes congestion, or the spilling of the fluid into the lungs and the accumulation of it in the feet. Even worse, adrenaline, which is released in response to lower blood pressure, causes the blood vessels to constrict, which makes it more difficult for the weakened heart to pump blood forward. Thus, a failing pump causes lower blood pressure, which leads to the release of hormones that cause constriction of the blood vessels and increased salt and water absorption; both of these make congestion worse and create a vicious cycle.

In recent years we've learned much about the hormones that are responsible for this vicious cycle. They are the same hormones that are released during stressful life events, and they are why stress can precipitate congestive heart failure in vulnerable patients. Drugs that are aimed at breaking up the congestion are designed specifically to block these hormones. Beta blockers, as they are called, are now touted as the most important drugs for treating congestive heart failure; they work by blocking the negative effects of adrenaline, and they help to break the vicious cycle. Angiotensin-converting enzyme (ACE) inhibitors block the effects of angiotensin, a potent vasoconstrictor, and diuretics remove the excess fluid caused by the antidiuretic hormone (ADH). Aldactone, an additional diuretic, works in part by blocking salt absorption.

Broken Pump: Improving Flow

The treatment for congestive heart failure involves a three-step plan to take the strain off the weakened heart muscle and ultimately improve the blood flow to the body's tissues.

Take a Load Off

The first step involves improving forward blood flow. This is accomplished by providing a path of least resistance. All fluid, including blood, will flow in the path of least resistance, making it easier for the weakened heart muscle to pump blood forward to the brain and the body.

The failure of the heart to contract forcefully causes the blood to back up like a congested highway. The solution is to widen the highway, adding a lane to improve forward traffic, and the medications for congestive heart failure are designed to do exactly that. By widening the highway or dilating the downstream blood vessels, we provide the path of least resistance and decrease the stress on the weakened heart; this leads to decreased congestion and improved forward blood flow. The term to describe this therapy is *afterload reduction*. Additional, nonpharmacological therapies for unloading the pump or providing the path of least resistance include ventricular assistance devices and balloon pumps.

Fluid Overload

The second step is to reduce the swelling that occurs when the heart becomes congested. During congestive heart failure, the heart becomes like an overfilled balloon, and the excess fluid spills off into the tissues, causing swelling of the face, the hands, the abdomen, and, because of gravity, especially the feet. This is similar to allowing a nightclub to fill with people beyond its capacity. If not monitored, an overcrowded nightclub can lead to a dangerous situation. As a responsible doorman keeps track of the maximum capacity in a nightclub, so too should a patient vulnerable to congestion monitor fluid intake. Because the weakened heart is always functioning close to capacity, one must be hypervigilant about monitoring fluid intake. I have found that patients with this condition do best when they know their ideal body weight and consume no more than 1.5 liters of fluid daily.

Digitalis is a drug that increases the force of contraction of the heart. It also slows the heart rate. According to a large trial, patients with cardiomyopathy (weakened heart muscle) and congestive heart failure who took digitalis had fewer symptoms, had fewer hospital admissions, and could exercise longer.

Surgery and Other Devices

The third step, in certain cases, involves surgery or the use of medical devices along with medications to further improve the function of the heart muscle.

Heart Transplants Heart transplantation, the ultimate surgical approach, is recommended only in patients for whom medications and devices don't help. Transplants have been shown to dramatically improve survival rates and the quality of life, but many patients have to wait a long time for a suitable donor. Fortunately, due to the effectiveness of therapy, some patients improve dramatically and are removed from the transplant lists.

ICD Some patients with cardiomyopathy and congestive heart failure have ticklish and irritable heart muscles that make their hearts prone to potentially life-threatening rhythms. An implantable cardioverter-defibrillator (ICD) is a pacemaker-like device that is implanted just under the skin, usually under the collarbone, which can detect these abnormal rhythms and provide a shock that corrects the rhythm.

In Sync   Up to 50 percent of patients with congestive heart failure have an abnormal electrical system, which makes the two bottom chambers of the heart beat in an uncoordinated fashion, further impairing the heart's pumping ability. They beat out of sequence, in an awkward, unsynchronized fashion. A newer therapy known as a biventricular (or both lower chambers) pacemaker sends an electrical impulse to both chambers simultaneously. This synchronizes their timing so that they contract in a more coordinated and efficient fashion.

Our Patient

Acting quickly, Amy's driver called 911, and within minutes an ambulance arrived at the scene, in the parking lot–like traffic, to tend to the patient. Amy was given oxygen and a potent fluid-removing diuretic intravenously. With lights flashing and sirens blaring, the ambulance rushed her to a nearby emergency room, where she died.

The required autopsy revealed a large heart, fluid in her lungs, and a severely weakened heart muscle; a special blood test proved that elevated pressure inside the heart was the likely cause of her congestion. The official reason for death was congestive heart failure due to medical and dietary noncompliance, exacerbated by emotional stress. The underlying chronic cause of the heart muscle's damage was long-standing, poorly controlled high blood pressure—one of the most common causes of this condition.

B - R - E - A - T - H - E
The Fallen Tree Exercise

This exercise is for people with a history of congestive heart failure.

Patients who have been admitted for congestive heart failure or who have a known cardiomyopathy will find this exercise to be very enjoyable and healing. I recommend that my patients practice each morning before taking their medications. Practicing regularly will help you to develop your relaxation skills and to train the neural connections between your brain and your heart. Stay focused and present. Notice your breathing and remember to concentrate on the simple concept of flow.

Focus and concentrate on the following three areas during the exercise:

1. Powerful source of flow
2. Fluid balance
3. Forward flow

Begin

Begin your exercise in your warm, cozy, and familiar place. Wear loose-fitting clothing and settle comfortably in your favorite chair or sofa. Always start your exercise by listening to the conversation. Remember that your heart and your brain are connected and in constant communication. Listen to your heart.

Take a deep breath in through your nose and let it out through your mouth. Count s-l-o-w-l-y to seven. Notice that when you take in a deep breath, your heart rate slightly increases, and as you exhale, your heart rate decreases. Take a few more breaths and notice this trend: in, your heart rate increases; out, your heart rate decreases. The more you practice, the better you will get at hearing your heartbeat. This is excellent proof that you are participating in the conversation.

As you begin, focus on your heart and clear your mind of any other thoughts. Liken this exercise to working out different muscles in the gym. Instead of working your back, your shoulders, or your biceps, look at this exercise as exercising and developing your heart-brain connection.

Relax

Remember that the relaxation response is a state of deep relaxation that is the opposite of the fight-or-flight response. You can reach this state by deep breathing. It is comfortable, soothing, and nurturing for your heart. Breathing in and out causes changes in the heart rate. When you take a deep breath in, you are activating the sympathetic nervous system, which causes your heart rate to speed up. When you exhale, count to seven, like the number of letters in B-R-E-A-T-H-E. This extended exhalation activates the parasympathetic nervous system and slows the heart rate by sending signals from your brain to your heart on a highway called the vagus nerve. This fluctuation or variability of the heart rate is good for the heart.

Envision

Visualize a river, gaze across it, and notice the majestic trees that line the shore. Observe that the trees are lined up together and that the gentle breeze causes them to sway synchronously and rhythmically.

Imagine that this synchronous rhythm is like your heart parts, with all the valves, arteries, and chambers working harmoniously together as an efficient pump propelling blood to all the tissues. Notice the warm sun on your shoulders and feel how this improves your circulation and your forward blood flow. Imagine that the flow of the river is constant and maintained by the strength and force of a waterfall. Notice how the water level and the depth of the river are maintained and constant, like your heart, in perfect balance.

Just upstream, closer to the waterfall that powers the river, you witness the falling of a large, broad-based tree. It falls gently, as if invisible hands were guiding it. As the tree approaches the surface of the river, you notice the roots as they come out of the ground and expose the nutritious soil, packed with minerals and fertile earth.

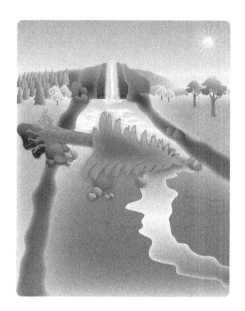
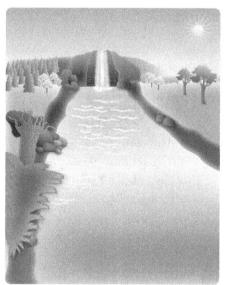

Once the tree has fallen into the water, it floats down the river, and you watch as it briefly stops and blocks the river. Unfazed by the obstruction, the waterfall powers through the transient impediment and pushes the huge tree out of its way. It happens so quickly that the depth of the river is unchanged. You make a mental note of this event and imagine that the strength of the waterfall and the powerful river flowing forward are like your heart pumping blood forward. Imagine that the almost effortless though powerful movement of the waterfall prevents the tree from obstruction; it is like the path of least resistance, providing smooth effortless flow to your brain and your body. It is like the powerful and smooth forward flow of the blood in your heart. It takes the path of least resistance and flows perfectly through open, smooth, and unimpeded blood vessels.

Apply

Make a mental connection and apply the image of a wide, smooth path to your blood vessels. Imagine that the trees you pass resemble healthy arteries and a smoothly flowing electrical system. Note that the beautiful vegetation around you represents your healthy heart. Listen to the sounds around you: the gentle breeze blowing in the trees, the chirping of the birds, and the sound of the distant waterfall resemble your heart—constant, rhythmic, and powerful.

Treat

View this exercise as a special treatment for yourself. You are deserving of this pleasurable and therapeutic time. The exercise is pleasurable, relaxing, and rejuvenating. This is not a chore or a task. Before long you will look forward to this work and feel like a runner who experiences a high from running.

Remember that this exercise, when performed correctly, is therapeutic and serves to decrease your heart rate, lower your blood pressure, and lower your vascular tone. The deeper and more relaxed you become, the more protective and effective is the therapy. Meditation and exercises such as B-R-E-A-T-H-E technique are therapeutic: they lower the levels of cardio-toxic hormones such as cortisol and adrenaline. This exercise increases heart-rate variability and low fluctuations in heart rate (low heart-rate variability) in patients who have been diagnosed with poor cardiovascular outcomes. Recall that guided imagery bolsters the immune system, lowers blood pressure and heart rate, and decreases anxiety.

Heal

When using the B-R-E-A-T-H-E technique, imagine the healing properties of relaxation. Your deep breathing helps you to train the nerves that connect the brain and the heart and has a calming and slowing effect on your heart rate. This exercise will reduce stress and make you feel better, which will enhance healing in your body. It will allow you to downshift so that your engine can cool and idle for a while. Imagine that the warm sun on your shoulders causes your blood vessels to dilate, further improving flow and thus healing your electrical system. Store the heart-healing metaphors in your memory so they can be quickly retrieved to help protect and heal your heart in a stressful situation.

End

As you end your B-R-E-A-T-H-E exercise, recall all of the heart-healing metaphors and summarize their significance and their relationship to your healing heart. Remember the perfectly flowing river, the beautiful swaying trees, and the powerful waterfall. Recall the powerful river as it gently sweeps the tree to the shore. As you end your exercise, you will become aware of your surroundings and feel energized. Your heart is strong, rhythmic, and unobstructed like the river.

4

Treating and Preventing
Heart Attacks

Dr. Charles Kimball appeared to be at the apex of his life. At forty-four, he had a thriving medical practice, a wonderful wife, and three healthy children. With a thick shock of auburn hair graying slightly at the temples and a healthy glow from regular and rigorous exercise, he was the picture of health and vitality. Nevertheless, the old saying that things are seldom as they appear turned out to be true for Dr. Kimball. One day, too much happened for his heart to handle.

He had gotten up early and knew he'd be lucky to be home before dark. He and his wife began their morning continuing an argument from the night before (which he knew was happening too frequently) about their teenage daughter, whose school grades had inexplicably fallen. His schedule was jammed with morning procedures (he silently prayed they'd all be routine) and more afternoon office visits than he could hope to handle.

Throughout the day, each time he managed a glance at his desk piled with foot-thick stacks of paper, the annoying case of heartburn he'd been hoping would go away ratcheted up a notch. He was in an examination room, explaining an upcoming cardiac procedure and trying to offer reassurance to a clearly terrified elderly male patient and his wife, when his assistant knocked on the door and asked him to step outside for a moment. The look in her eyes signaled that something was wrong. Promising a quick return, he excused himself, closed the door behind him, and heard his assistant say, "It's something about your father; your sister is on the phone in your office." As Dr. Kimball strode nervously down the corridor, he wondered what could possibly be wrong with his father. After all, his dad, who also happened to be his best friend, was the healthiest sixty-nine-year-old on the planet.

His sister's first words, "Dad has had a massive stroke, and they're saying he might not make it," were like a stinging slap across his face. The rest of the words were only a jumble: "You have to fly here right now. Mom says she doesn't want to live if Dad doesn't make it" and a hysterical "Can't you do something? You're a doctor!" As he tried to calm his sister down and learn as much as he could about what had happened and what the doctors were doing, he glanced toward his office door and saw his assistant trying to get his attention, then he heard his pager buzz wildly. One look at the message on it, as well as the look on his assistant's face, told him what was happening: a patient from a morning procedure was in critical condition, and he was needed immediately.

He told his sister that he was in the middle of a medical emergency and would call back as soon as possible, asked his assistant to explain his absence to the patient he had just been talking to, and started mentally reviewing as many details as he could remember about the condition of the patient from the morning procedure.

The distance between his medical office and the hospital was only a quarter mile, but the faster he walked, the greater the distance seemed to become. His mind was racing. He had a patient in trouble; his father was having a stroke; his wife was angry and disappointed; his sister was hysterical. What should he do first? As he approached the hospital's back-door doctor's entrance, he braced himself for the four flights of stairs and decided to run up them. He'd fix the immediate problem first, then deal with everything else. After all, he fixed things for a living.

Dr. Kimball didn't get to see and help his patient that day, although he did make it to the intensive care unit. Halfway up the stairs he tore his left anterior descending artery and suffered a massive heart attack. I was the cardiologist who was called in to help save Dr. Kimball's life.

CARDIOLOGIST'S ANALYSIS
Torn

Some form of heart attack will strike nearly a million people in the United States each year. Two-thirds of all people who have one won't have experienced any previous symptoms, and one's sex doesn't grant immunity: heart attacks are an equal opportunity foe of both men and women.

The classic story you just read illustrates how a stressful life event can precipitate a fatal or nearly fatal cardiac event. Dr. Kimball is *torn*, having to deal with two emergencies at once. The stress is overwhelming and creates a sudden flooding of toxic hormones, which causes his coronary artery to *tear*, leading to a massive heart attack.

Don't Be Burned by Heartburn

In my practice I've observed that people typically experience a pattern of both psychological and physical changes during a cardiac event.

Symptoms of chest discomfort are often mistakenly attributed to an upset stomach, acid reflux, or gas. This misdiagnosis and minimizing of symptoms is part denial, "this can't be my heart," and part reality, because the heart, the esophagus (swallowing tube), and the stomach are in close proximity to one another.

The two organs most commonly affected by stress are the stomach and the heart. In a recent survey, more than 50 percent of heartburn episodes were linked to stress. This is why the diagnosis of cardiac chest pain versus acid reflux is a common pitfall.

My strong advice is that if you have heartburn, you should first consider the "burning" as arising from your heart instead of your stomach. Seek professional help, and if it turns out to be your stomach, good for you! I've seen the reverse situation too many times, in which people ignore and minimize heartburn and miss an incredible lifesaving opportunity.

The Pain before a Heart Attack

The stuttering pain that some people experience prior to a heart attack is known as *angina pectoris*, which is Latin for "pain in the chest." Over time the artery develops a buildup of debris called plaque that partially obstructs the flow and starves the heart muscle of oxygen.

Similar to an infant who cries when hungry, the heart is thirsty for blood and cries out for nourishment by manifesting chest pain. Pain from heart disease varies widely. Some people have nausea, neck pain, back pain, jaw pain, or even arm pain as the warning sign of a heart attack.

Yet, ironically, most people have no warning signs whatsoever of an imminent heart attack. This is why symptoms should be regarded as helpful signals sent from a heart in distress. Consider yourself fortunate if you experience them. Any bodily clues should be regarded as extremely important and possibly even lifesaving.

Dr. Kimball illustrates the denial that is commonly seen in patients who are in the throes of a threatening heart attack. He mistakenly chose to ignore the symptoms and attributed them to heartburn. Little was he willing to realize that these symptoms were red flags that should have been heeded. A dynamic process inside his coronary artery was occurring, and his symptoms represented a bomb threatening to detonate.

The Clogged Pipe: Blood Clots

In Dr. Kimball's case, stress triggered a contained mini-explosion within his coronary artery. The sudden change in blood pressure and heart rate caused by the flooding of adrenaline and cortisol caused an increase in the stress in the artery wall, leading to a local tear or rupture.

Blood vessels are also weakened by inflammation. The part of the plaque that is especially prone to tear is known as the shoulder. In this region of the plaque, research has found high concentrations of immune cells that release destructive enzymes, which weaken the plaque and link inflammation to plaque rupture.

These complications are chronic, slowly progressive, and cumulative. Soft plaque usually ruptures suddenly, causing the formation of a thrombus (a clot of blood that forms within a blood vessel and remains attached to its place of origin). The thrombus will rapidly slow or stop the blood flow (often within five minutes or less) through the coronary artery, leading to death of the tissues fed by the artery.

The mini-explosion inside Dr. Kimball's blood vessel led to a cascade of events that caused his blood to become thick, sticky, and prone to clot. Responding to a tear in the vessel wall, his body summoned his clotting system to repair the broken vessel.

Thrombosis, as this condition is called, is similar to what happens when you apply pressure on a minor cut: a clot forms, and the bleeding stops. When the blood vessel is completely blocked, the heart muscle begins to die. This event is called a myocardial infarction.

Unfortunately, blood clotting inside a coronary artery is problematic, because although it may fix the tear in the blood vessel, it clogs the pipe and obstructs the blood flow. This is known as coronary thrombosis. The blood supply to the heart muscle, now cut off, starves the heart muscle of oxygen and causes part of the heart to die—the process known as a heart attack.

Restoring Flow

If the situation is recognized quickly, restoring blood flow to the damaged artery can minimize and sometimes completely avoid heart damage; it's like dodging a bullet. In an emergency situation, when a coronary artery is 100 percent blocked, we know that the optimal therapy is a stent procedure to relieve the obstruction. In other situations, coronary artery bypass grafting (CABG, pronounced "cabbage") and medications are used to restore the blood flow to the thirsty heart muscle. Each of these therapeutic options is described below.

Lose the Waist: Angioplasty and Stents

Doctors describe blockages in the coronary artery as being like an hourglass, an apple core, or a napkin ring. Common to all of these descriptions is a central narrowing, or "waist." In the cardiac catheterization laboratory, where blocked arteries are repaired through angioplasty and stenting, the term *losing the waist* is used to mean expanding the narrow space. Stents, small metal tubes that provide scaffolding and reinforcement for the damaged blood vessel, have been shown to be the best therapy for treating heart attacks. They resemble the small spring in a ballpoint pen. Positioned at the site of the blockage, the stent is pressed against the walls of the blood vessel under pressure, immediately allowing the blood vessel to fully open so that blood flow can be restored. For optimal results, this procedure should be performed within ninety minutes of the patient's arrival at the hospital.

An Alternative Route: Bypass Surgery

Coronary bypass surgery creates a new pathway or an alternative route for blood flow around the blocked artery, allowing blood to reach the heart muscle again. A healthy blood vessel from either your leg or your chest wall is used to restore blood flow. If you have multiple blockages, then more than one bypass is used.

CABG is the most commonly performed major operation in the world. Last year more than five hundred thousand CABG operations were performed in the United States. This operation is offered to patients when stenting isn't possible.

The Heart, Stress, and Drugs

Medications that have been proven to prevent heart attacks include aspirin, beta blockers, statins, and angiotensin-converting enzyme (ACE) inhibitors. Each of these drugs blocks at least one of the negative effects of stress, which has been shown to increase heart rate, blood pressure, inflammation, constriction of the blood vessels, and inflammation.

Aspirin is a potent blocker of blood clots and a potent anti-inflammatory. Beta blockers blunt the effect of adrenaline and lower heart rate and blood pressure. ACE inhibitors lower blood pressure and decrease constriction of blood vessels. Statins decrease coronary remodeling, or buildup of plaque in the arterial wall. Coronary remodeling refers to changes in the arterial wall due to atherosclerosis. Early in the disease process as plaque accumulates (and is deposited in the vessel wall), the artery dilates or increases in size in a process known as "positive remodeling." Later in the disease, the plaque matures and forms a scar that makes the blood vessel smaller and constrict, known as "negative remodeling."

The data show that these drugs decrease the risk of heart attack and stroke by up to 30 percent. If you have risk factors such as high blood pressure, high cholesterol, diabetes, a family history of premature coronary artery disease, or tobacco use, you should discuss the possibility of taking these drugs with your physician, always weighing the benefits against the risk of potential side effects. This is the most important point about prevention. Successful prevention involves identifying those who are asymptomatic though at risk and stand to benefit most from treatment.

The Body's Natural Bypass: Collaterals

Coronary collaterals are natural bypasses—alternative sources of blood supply that the body forms in response to a blocked artery. Some patients have heart attacks but never lose any heart muscle function due to the development of these amazing natural bypass vessels. Unfortunately, not everyone has the ability to form collaterals. Large collateral arteries are present in up to one-third of patients with coronary artery disease.

Our Patient

Dr. Kimball underwent the emergency stenting of his left anterior descending artery—referred to by doctors as the "widow maker"—and his life was saved.

When I spoke with him in the ICU after the procedure, he remained incredulous about what had happened and spoke the same words I've heard thousands of times: "I eat right, and I exercise. How could this have happened to me? What more could I have done?"

I told him about a series of exercises that could have helped him tremendously and maybe even have prevented his heart attack. It's sad but true that most people are ready to take preventive measures only after they have already been traumatized by a major upheaval or crisis. Such was the case with this patient; now he was ready and willing to listen and learn.

Many months after his cardiac event, I saw Dr. Kimball at the scrub sink, seemingly preoccupied. I greeted him and asked how he was doing. He told me that he uses his time at the sink to do his B-R-E-A-T-H-E exercises, and he added that since he started using the techniques I'd taught him, he's never felt better. He said he feels focused, relaxed, and in control. Then he gave me a big knowing smile and asked the question I've been asked so many times before. "Doc," he said, "why didn't I start doing these exercises a lot earlier?"

Flow with It

In medical school, doctors are taught that blood flows through the body in a process known as fluid dynamics, and they study the motion of the fluid and how it moves through a tube.

The flow of any liquid can be smooth, consistent, and unobstructed, like the flow of a beautiful river. This calm, free flow is known as *laminar*. On the other hand, the flow can be fast, erratic, and chaotic, with wild twists and turns and tortuous whitewater rapids.

The heart that is working efficiently has a smooth laminar flow, and the heart that is weak has a turbulent flow. The B-R-E-A-T-H-E technique enables you to tame the river of the heart and to successfully navigate or avoid the stressful turbulent rapids in life. You will be able to flow freely through the river, reaching your destination safely and calmly.

The entire workings of the heart can be simplified to a single concept: flow. The coronary arteries require adequate flow to provide the heart muscle with blood; the valves, or the doors that connect the chambers, are controlled by forward flow; and the electrical system requires the flow of an electrical current from top to bottom to cause the heart to contract.

It follows, then, that healing metaphors for the heart should involve the simple concept of *flow*. Galen, the ancient Greek physician, was an incredible visionary. He was completely accurate with his concepts of pneuma (breath) and the relationship between the heart and the brain. He was also extremely perceptive in his use of the river metaphor to describe the heart and the vascular system.

The cardiovascular system is a fluid-filled container composed of a series of long winding tubes, some large (like the Mississippi or the Nile River) and some small (like tiny brooks, creeks, or rivulets). The river, which novelists and poets for centuries after Galen have used as a symbol for life, will serve as the primary metaphor in the heart-healing exercises that follow.

The flow of the river is like the pattern of life: sometimes smooth, calm, and serene and sometimes turbulent, fast, curvy, and unpredictable. The river is alive, breathing, and dependent on the changes of the seasons. In winter, the river water is cold, the level is high, and the flow is rapid. In the summer the water is warm, the level is low, and the flow is slower.

Like the heart, the river has a circulation system. It collects water from mountain runoff, streams, and creeks to form a single artery that delivers its contents to the waterfall, which acts like the heart, providing the power source for the downstream flow of the river. The water flows from the waterfall to the river, which acts like the arterial system, delivering water to wildlife and vegetation. This is similar to the heart's arterial system, which delivers blood to the vital organs.

This cycle of the river, which maintains a continuous flow, is much like your cardiovascular system, which collects blood and then delivers it in a constant rhythmic pattern. The river, like life, has rapids, which act like stress: fast, unpredictable, and turbulent.

The tools in this book will be the rudder in your boat to help you navigate the rapids and enable you to predict what's around the bend. Ultimately, you will learn to B-R-E-AT-H-E through the rapids so you can maximize the time spent in the calm section of the river, which will protect your heart and maintain the flow.

Just as an athlete imagines a perfect shot and then executes it, and just as an opera singer imagines singing a perfect aria and then performs it, you will learn to B-R-E-A-T-H-E and begin to experience a heart that flows, like the river, powerful and strong.

B-R-E-A-T-H-E
The River Exercise

This exercise is for those with existing coronary artery disease. Patients who have had angioplasty, stents, or bypass surgery will find this exercise useful, relaxing, and extremely pleasurable. If you have not had coronary artery disease but wish to prevent it, go on to the next section.

When doing this exercise, use the techniques described to help you develop a uniform and consistent practice. Practicing regularly, like toning your muscles in the gym, will help you to develop relaxation skills and to train the neural connections between your brain and your heart. Throughout the exercise, focus on the heart-healing metaphors; note how the symbols are curative and relate to your heart.

Begin

Begin your exercise in your warm, cozy, and familiar place. Wear loose-fitting clothing and settle comfortably in your favorite chair or sofa. Always start your exercise by listening to the conversation. Remember that your heart and your brain are connected and in constant communication. Listen to your heart.

Take a deep breath in through your nose and let it out through your mouth. Count s-l-o-w-l-y to seven. Notice that when you take in a deep breath, your heart rate slightly increases, and as you exhale, your heart rate decreases. Take a few more breaths and notice this trend: in, your heart rate increases; out, your heart rate decreases. The more you practice, the better you will get at hearing your heartbeat. This is excellent proof that you are participating in the conversation.

As you begin, focus on your heart and clear your mind of any other thoughts. Liken this exercise to working out different muscles in the gym. Instead of working your back, your shoulders, or your biceps, look at this exercise as exercising and developing your heart-brain connection.

Relax

Remember that the relaxation response is a state of deep relaxation that is the opposite of the fight-or-flight response. You can reach this state by deep breathing. It is comfortable, soothing, and nurturing for your heart. Breathing in and out causes changes in the heart rate. When you take a deep breath in, you are activating the sympathetic nervous system, which causes your heart rate to speed up. When you exhale, count to seven, like the number of letters in B-R-E-A-T-H-E. This extended exhalation activates the parasympathetic nervous system and slows the heart rate by sending signals from your brain to your heart on a highway called the vagus nerve. This fluctuation or variability of the heart rate is good for the heart.

Envision

Pay special attention to the slate-lined banks of a beautiful flowing river, the new rivulets and water channels forming in front of you, the new growth that forms from the flow of the water, and the powerful rhythmic flow of the river. Notice that a constant flow is generated by the majestic waterfall in the distance. Feel the warm sun on your shoulders and think of how the clean, crystal-clear water is the life source for all of the beautiful vegetation and wildlife around you. Make a mental note as you focus on each of the metaphors described in the exercise. Note the new rivulets and channels of flow created by the majestic river. Imagine the stability and strength of the banks of the river and how the flow is contained and directed perfectly within them.

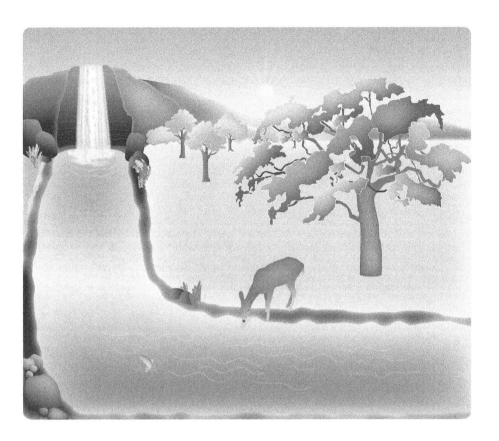

Apply

Make a mental connection and apply how the smooth, slate-lined banks of the river are like the strong and sturdy walls of your reinforced and stented blood vessels. Imagine how the new rivulets and tributaries resemble new arterial growth and how the new sprouting and flowering vegetation represents new healthy heart muscle. Imagine how the waterfall, the power source, maintains the constant flow of the river and how this resembles your heart: constant, rhythmic, and powerful. Observe the massive tree that shades the river, and think of its thick, solid, multiringed base and how this is similar to the strong, stable walls of your coronary arteries.

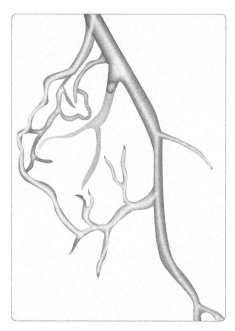 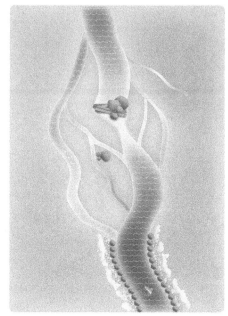

Treat

View this exercise as a special treatment for yourself. You are deserving of this pleasurable and therapeutic time. The exercise is pleasurable, relaxing, and rejuvenating. This is not a chore or a task. Before long you will look forward to this work and feel like a runner who experiences a high from running.

Remember that this exercise, when performed correctly, is therapeutic and serves to decrease your heart rate, lower your blood pressure, and lower your vascular tone. The deeper and more relaxed you become, the more protective and effective is the therapy. Meditation and exercises such as B-R-E-A-T-H-E technique are therapeutic: they lower the levels of cardio-toxic hormones such as cortisol and adrenaline. This exercise increases heart-rate variability and low fluctuations in heart rate (low heart-rate variability) in patients who have been diagnosed with poor cardiovascular outcomes. Recall that guided imagery bolsters the immune system, lowers blood pressure and heart rate, and decreases anxiety.

Heal

When using the B-R-E-A-T-H-E technique, imagine the healing properties of relaxation. Your deep breathing helps you to train the nerves that connect the brain and the heart and has a calming and slowing effect on your heart rate. This exercise will reduce stress and make you feel better, which will enhance healing in your body. It will allow you to downshift so that your engine can cool and idle for a while. Imagine that the warm sun on your shoulders causes your blood vessels to dilate, further improving flow and thus healing your electrical system. Store the heart-healing metaphors in your memory so they can be quickly retrieved to help protect and heal your heart in a stressful situation.

End

As you end your B-R-E-A-T-H-E exercise, recall all of the heart-healing metaphors and summarize their significance and their relationship to your healing heart. Remember the perfectly flowing river, the beautiful swaying trees, and the powerful waterfall. Recall the powerful river as it gently sweeps the tree to the shore. As you end your exercise, you will become aware of your surroundings and feel energized. Your heart is strong, rhythmic, and unobstructed like the river.

B-R-E-A-T-H-E

The Path of Relaxation

This exercise is designed to prevent coronary artery disease by decreasing stress. It is also extremely beneficial for reducing stress for the spouse, family, and other loved ones of someone who has recently experienced a cardiac event. You and your cardiovascular system will thoroughly enjoy and appreciate this heart-healing exercise.

Use the B-R-E-A-T-H-E technique and apply the heart-healing metaphors to your heart. As you read along and focus on the sights, sounds, and feelings, recall the teaching points about coronary artery disease outlined in the cardiologist's analysis.

Remember to focus on reversing the coronary remodeling process, and imagine the walls of your arteries as stable and strong.

To the spouse, family member, or loved one of a heart patient, I recommend reading the exercise above, for those with coronary artery disease. It will broaden your understanding of the disease and help with providing empathy, compassion, and support, which are all essential for protecting and healing our hearts.

Begin

Begin your exercise in your warm, cozy, and familiar place. Wear loose-fitting clothing and settle comfortably in your favorite chair or sofa. Always start your exercise by listening to the conversation. Remember that your heart and your brain are connected and in constant communication. Listen to your heart.

Take a deep breath in through your nose and let it out through your mouth. Count s-l-o-w-l-y to seven. Notice that when you take in a deep breath, your heart rate slightly increases, and as you exhale, your heart rate decreases. Take a few more breaths and notice this trend: in, your heart rate increases; out, your heart rate decreases. The more you practice, the better you will get at hearing your heartbeat. This is excellent proof that you are participating in the conversation.

As you begin, focus on your heart and clear your mind of any other thoughts. Liken this exercise to working out different muscles in the gym. Instead of working your back, your shoulders, or your biceps, look at this exercise as exercising and developing your heart-brain connection.

Relax

Remember that the relaxation response is a state of deep relaxation that is the opposite of the fight-or-flight response. You can reach this state by deep breathing. It is comfortable, soothing, and nurturing for your heart. Breathing in and out causes changes in the heart rate. When you take a deep breath in, you are activating the sympathetic nervous system, which causes your heart rate to speed up. When you exhale, count to seven, like the number of letters in B-R-E-A-T-H-E. This extended exhalation activates the parasympathetic nervous system and slows the heart rate by sending signals from your brain to your heart on a highway called the vagus nerve. This fluctuation or variability of the heart rate is good for the heart.

Envision

Imagine a beautiful hiking trail. It is very familiar to you. You recognize the sights, the smells, and the sounds. It reminds you of a pleasurable experience from childhood. You feel warm, comfortable, and relaxed.

The trail is marked by walking stones that guide and draw you forward, and with each step you feel more and more relaxed. You are breathing in through your nose and out through your mouth. You are deeply relaxed, yet alert, and keenly aware of the sights and sounds around you.

You feel the connection between your heart rate and your breathing, and hear the conversation.

The trail is clearly demarcated, lined by beautiful evergreen trees. It consists of red adobe dust that is soft on your feet like fine, smooth powder. You feel drawn to the end of the trail, where you see a flickering light caused by the sun's reflection on the water and hear a strong roar of running water.

The end of the trail transitions from tall evergreen trees to knee-high grassy shrubbery, which gives way to a lime-green mossy perch at the foot of the majestic river. As you approach

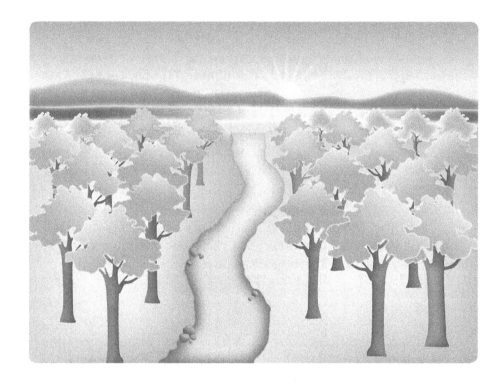

the end of the trail, you sense a strong welcoming feeling. You feel as though you were invited to enjoy this beautiful, serene, and calm place—a place to worship and heal your heart.

Apply

Make a mental connection and apply the image of a wide, smooth path to your blood vessels. Imagine that the trees you pass resemble healthy arteries and a smoothly flowing electrical system. Note that the beautiful vegetation around you represents your healthy heart. Listen to the sounds around you: the gentle breeze blowing in the trees, the chirping of the birds, and the sound of the distant waterfall resemble your heart—constant, rhythmic and powerful.

Treat

View this exercise as a special treatment for yourself. You are deserving of this pleasurable and therapeutic time. The exercise is pleasurable, relaxing, and rejuvenating. This is not a chore or a task. Before long you will look forward to this work and feel like a runner who experiences a high from running.

Remember that this exercise, when performed correctly, is therapeutic and serves to decrease your heart rate, lower your blood pressure, and lower your vascular tone. The deeper and more relaxed you become, the more protective and effective is the therapy. Meditation and exercises such as B-R-E-A-T-H-E technique are therapeutic: they lower the levels of cardio-toxic hormones such as cortisol and adrenaline. This exercise increases heart-rate variability and low fluctuations in heart rate (low heart-rate variability) in patients who have been diagnosed with poor cardiovascular outcomes. Recall that guided imagery bolsters the immune system, lowers blood pressure and heart rate, and decreases anxiety.

Heal

When using the B-R-E-A-T-H-E technique, imagine the healing properties of relaxation. Your deep breathing helps you to train the nerves that connect the brain and the heart and has a calming and slowing effect on your heart rate. This exercise will reduce stress and make you feel better, which will enhance healing in your body. It will allow you to downshift so that your engine can cool and idle for a while. Imagine that the warm sun on your shoulders causes your blood vessels to dilate, further improving flow and thus healing your electrical system. Store the heart-healing metaphors in your memory so they can be quickly retrieved to help protect and heal your heart in a stressful situation.

End

As you end your B-R-E-A-T-H-E exercise, recall all of the heart-healing metaphors and summarize their significance and their relationship to your healing heart. Remember the perfectly flowing river, the beautiful swaying trees, and the powerful waterfall. Recall the powerful river as it gently sweeps the tree to the shore. As you end your exercise, you will become aware of your surroundings and feel energized. Your heart is strong, rhythmic, and unobstructed like the river.

5

Treating and Preventing Arrhythmias

Sally Jones, age fifty-four, comes from a long line of teachers. Her mother taught elementary school for forty years, and almost all of her aunts were teachers. They, like she, believed teaching to be a noble profession whose rewards included respect in the community and a reliable income in retirement.

Most of all, Miss Jones (as she likes to be called) loved her inner-city students at Harris Elementary School. During the twenty-six years she'd been teaching either third or fourth grade, more than seven hundred students had passed through her classroom, and she was proud of the fact that she could remember every student's name and something about him or her.

During her entire teaching career, Miss Jones's guiding principle was that if children were taught to read, write, do math, and act with proper manners, they would become productive and fulfilled members of society. She was a strict, no-nonsense teacher, but her style was magnetic, and one of her great joys in life was the hundreds of thank-you letters and holiday cards she'd received from former students and their parents. The oversized scrapbooks in which she saved each of her treasures defined her being.

The past year had been extremely difficult. Her mother had passed away after a long, painful bout of cancer. The gentlemen friend she'd had for years had suddenly decided that he was no longer interested in a relationship with her, and he was now involved with a fellow choir member twenty-five years her junior. Miss Jones felt constantly tired, and no matter how much sleeping she did at night or on the weekend, she couldn't shake her sense of exhaustion.

Her eating habits had suffered as well. After years of cooking for her ill mother and her male friend, she was almost relieved not to have to cook, and she had resorted to TV dinners at night and snack foods from the vending machines in the teacher's lounge for her lunches. In the past year her weight had ballooned from the 185 pounds that she'd always carried well to somewhere over the 200-pound mark.

In addition to all of this, Miss Jones began having severe headaches, which she attributed to her frequent sinus infections and for which she took over-the-counter decongestants, but they did not seem to help.

Her biggest health concern was what was happening with her heart. It had recently started racing out of control for seemingly no reason, and this would be accompanied by sheer panic. It always went away after a few minutes, however, so she fought desperately to ignore these warning signs and hoped that they would not return.

On the outside, Miss Jones appeared calm and collected, but on the inside she was fighting to maintain that image and was fast becoming a nervous wreck because she was worrying herself sick.

Each day seemed to bring more trouble. The previous week, the school board had announced the certainty of more teacher layoffs for the upcoming year, and she started believing (despite her seniority and her sterling reputation) that she'd be the next to go. Her school's test scores were among the worst in the school district, despite her hard work, and it seemed as though the students and the parents had lost all respect for the teachers. Just two days earlier an unruly student had hurled a book at her, shouted an obscenity at her, and marched out of class. The student's parents had blamed her for their child's behavior.

Miss Jones had started showing up late for teachers' meetings, and on two occasions she had simply forgotten about them. Her school administrator tried talking to her about the changes in her weight, her attitude, and her behavior, but she simply shrugged off his attempts by citing a heavy workload and her worries about the students.

One day in late May, an hour after the students had been dismissed for the day, Miss Jones was sitting at her desk surrounded by piles of uncorrected papers when the seldomly used school telephone on the wall close to her desk issued a shrill ring. It startled her. She stood up, walked several feet to the telephone, glanced at the caller ID, and saw that it was the school principal calling. She was convinced that he was calling to tell her she was being laid off, and she became panic-stricken.

Immediately Miss Jones felt palpitations in her chest, became short of breath, and felt a strange tingling in her right arm. She anxiously tried to reach out for the phone, but her right arm failed to cooperate and hung lazily next to her like a rag doll. When she finally lifted the phone with her left hand and clumsily held the receiver next to her ear, she started to say something but was unable to speak. She knew that something was terribly wrong, so with her last bit of resolve, she hung up and then called 911.

When the paramedics arrived, Miss Jones was lying across her desk on top of her ungraded vocabulary tests. Her right side was noticeably weak, and her speech was garbled but understandable as she explained to the medics what had transpired.

She was brought to a nearby emergency room, where an electrocardiogram revealed atrial fibrillation, or irregular heart rhythm. Her pulse rate was 180 beats per minute, and her blood pressure was 200/90. She was treated intravenously with a drug to control her heart rate, and it worked almost instantaneously. A head computerized tomography (CT) scan and blood tests were ordered, and she was admitted to the hospital. After a number of other studies and a visit with a neurologist and a cardiologist, she was discharged with the diagnosis of atrial fibrillation from hypertensive heart disease complicated by stroke.

Before her discharge from the hospital, a meeting with her doctors was scheduled. Her internist, her cardiologist, and her neurologist all expressed their concern about the direct relationship of her work stress to the onset of her arrhythmia and stroke, and they strongly recommended that she somehow modify the pressures in her workplace.

Just twelve months later, thirty pounds lighter, and full of vigor, Miss Jones was voted Teacher of the Year. She attributed her successful turnaround to the B-R-E-A-T-H-E technique, which she performs regularly before her daily two-mile hike along the Potomac River just outside her classroom. She especially enjoys the beautiful cherry trees that line the sides of the majestic river.

CARDIOLOGIST'S ANALYSIS
Out of Rhythm and the Blues

Miss Jones represents a classic example of someone with atrial fibrillation, an erratic heart rhythm that affects 2 million Americans and 4.5 million Europeans.

When atrial fibrillation occurs, the heart's electrical system begins firing erratically and irregularly. Although it's not usually life-threatening. this arrhythmia can be extremely uncomfortable and, if unrecognized, can lead to a debilitating stroke.

Atrial fibrillation occurs when the top two chambers of the heart quiver and beat at 375–400 beats per minute. The bottom chambers of the heart, known as the ventricles, are capable of beating only half as fast, 175–200 beats per minute, which correlates with a rapid pulse and a feeling of pounding in the chest. When the top chambers quiver, or fibrillate, the blood in these chambers becomes stagnant and prone to clot. The clot can break off and travel from the heart to the brain, causing a stroke.

Fearing job loss, Miss Jones became anxious and depressed. This weakened her immune system and led to repeated sinus infections. She unknowingly made matters worse by taking over-the-counter decongestants, which are common culprits for causing an irregular heart rhythm.

Consumed by the pressures of work, she became socially isolated and developed maladaptive cravings for foods that are high in fat and sugar content. Complicating the situation, she became dehydrated, which caused the stress hormone adrenaline to rise even more.

Work stress led to depression and a weakened immune system, which caused recurrent infections. This led to atrial fibrillation, causing a clot to form and break off; it traveled from her heart to her brain and caused a stroke. The patients who are at the highest risk for blood clots and a stroke are typically at least seventy years old, hypertensive, and diabetic, with a previous history of stroke and congestive heart failure.

The quivering chambers and the resulting irregular, erratic pulse also cause the following symptoms:

- Dizziness
- Palpitations
- Weakness
- Fatigue
- Shortness of breath

- Stroke
- Chest pain

Worried Sick: Stress, Palpitations, and Panic

Panic attacks, like the one Miss Jones experienced, are associated with heart disease, particularly in women. A recent study showed that women who reported at least one panic attack were at higher risk of having cardiovascular illness and death after an average of five years of follow-up.

Stress can precipitate panic attacks, which lead to the release of adrenaline, which in turn causes abnormal electrical impulses and arrhythmias.

The causes of atrial fibrillation are numerous, but the most common include the following:

- Emotional stress
- High levels of the thyroid hormone
- Excess alcohol
- Pneumonia
- Coronary artery disease
- High blood pressure
- Heart surgery
- Stimulant drugs, which include nasal decongestants, caffeine, nicotine, cocaine, and amphetamines (including diet pills)

Diagnosing and Treating Atrial Fibrillation

To reach a diagnosis of atrial fibrillation, the doctor asks a number of important questions. A thorough physical exam is performed, followed by a series of tests that will confirm the diagnosis. Initial tests include an ECG, a chest X-ray, and an echocardiogram (or echo). A chest X-ray will indicate congestive heart failure or pneumonia. An ECG is a tracing of the electrical activity of the heart, and an echo is an ultrasound that reveals heart muscle function and the workings of the valves. Blood samples are collected in order to look for markers that indicate heart muscle damage, heart attack, and thyroid hormone levels. There are many other tests, determined by the patient history, that can be used to help make the diagnosis.

The medications for atrial fibrillation are prescribed for three reasons: to slow the heart rate, to maintain a regular rhythm, and to thin the blood. The combination of medications prescribed for atrial fibrillation is determined by the risk of blood clots, the symptoms, and the cause.

Anticoagulation

Many patients with atrial fibrillation require a blood thinner, known as an anticoagulant, to prevent strokes. Certain risk factors, such as age (older than seventy), high blood pressure, diabetes, congestive heart failure, and a previous history of stroke all increase the risk of blood clot formation if you have atrial fibrillation.

Rate versus Rhythm

Rate-control medications slow the heart down and prevent it from beating too fast when atrial fibrillation occurs. Common drugs that control rate include digitalis, calcium channel blockers, and beta blockers. The medications that are used to maintain a regular rhythm and to help prevent recurrent episodes of atrial fibrillation are called anti-arrhythmics and include drugs such as sotalol and amiodarone. Anti-arrhythmic medications can be tricky and usually require a cardiologist to help manage dosage and to watch for potential side effects.

Ablation

For patients who have atrial fibrillation that is difficult to control or treat with medications, a procedure known as radio-frequency ablation may be considered. Ablation is a procedure in which a small, irritable, and arrhythmia-causing spot is destroyed or removed. A scar then forms and decreases the likelihood of the arrhythmia from recurring.

Maze

The maze procedure involves making a series of precise incisions in the top chambers of the heart (the atria) to interrupt the conduction of abnormal impulses. This allows rhythmic and regular impulses to travel normally through the cardiac electrical system.

Cardioversion

In some cases the doctor will attempt to get your heart back into a regular rhythm by "cardioverting." Cardioversion can be accomplished either with a small electrical shock or with medications. This should be performed only in certain situations; when it is done electively, it requires that your blood be appropriately thinned for three full weeks prior to the conversion.

B-R-E-A-T-H-E
The Cherry Blossom Exercise

This exercise is for treating and preventing arrhythmias, abnormal heart rhythms that are triggered by stress and are caused by a short circuit in the cardiac electrical system. There are a number of arrhythmias other than atrial fibrillation for which this exercise will be beneficial.

Imagine the perfect flow of an efficient cardiac electrical system. An electrical current begins in the top chambers and ends in the bottom chambers of the heart. The flow of electrical current through the heart's electrical system turns around and repeats itself, generating a consistent and forceful pulse.

So sit back, relax, and enjoy the ebb, flow, and pleasurable rhythm of the following exercise.

Begin

Begin your exercise in your warm, cozy, and familiar place. Wear loose-fitting clothing and settle comfortably in your favorite chair or sofa. Always start your exercise by listen ing to the conversation. Remember that your heart and your brain are connected and in constant communication. Listen to your heart.

Take a deep breath in through your nose and let it out through your mouth. Count s-l-o-w-l-y to seven. Notice that when you take in a deep breath, your heart rate slightly increases, and as you exhale, your heart rate decreases. Take a few more breaths and notice this trend: in, your heart rate increases; out, your heart rate decreases. The more you practice, the better you will get at hearing your heartbeat. This is excellent proof that you are participating in the conversation.

As you begin, focus on your heart and clear your mind of any other thoughts. Liken this exercise to working out different muscles in the gym. Instead of working your back, your shoulders, or your biceps, look at this exercise as exercising and developing your heart-brain connection.

Relax

Remember that the relaxation response is a state of deep relaxation that is the opposite of the fight-or-flight response. You can reach this state by deep breathing. It is comfortable, soothing, and nurturing for your heart. Breathing in and out causes changes in the heart rate. When you take a deep breath in, you are activating the sympathetic nervous system, which causes your heart rate to speed up. As you exhale, count to seven, like the number of letters in B-R-E-A-T-H-E. This extended exhalation activates the parasympathetic nervous system and slows the heart rate by sending signals from your brain to your heart on a highway called the vagus nerve. This fluctuation or variability of the heart rate is good for the heart.

Envision

Imagine sitting at the foot of a river and noticing over your shoulder the branch of a cherry tree.

You marvel over a beautiful cherry blossom at its tip, covered by the mist from the nearby waterfall. Its colors are vivid: deep pink and white on the background of a deep, rich, cherrywood stem.

The branch is hanging perfectly, as if it were purposefully placed just over a small inlet from the majestic river.

The blossom is drenched in the crisp, clear, iridescent mist, which drips rhythmically onto the glasslike water beneath. You

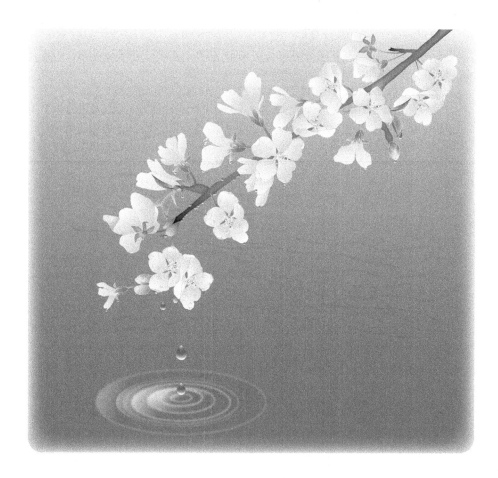

notice the rhythm and cadence of the droplets—one each second.

Constant and perfectly predictable each droplet falls, and you observe a cycle that starts from the waterfall's mist. First, the branch becomes saturated with mist. Next, the branch collects the crystal-clear water, which then flows to the end of the branch, where the water accumulates and forms a droplet. Finally, the droplet falls and enters the water below, creating a gentle wave across the inlet. This repetitious pattern and rhythm is soothing and mesmerizing.

Each drop is perfectly formed by mist sprayed from the powerful source. As each drop touches the surface below, small ringlets form, which move gently across the inlet to the river's edge. You begin to hear and feel your heart. Soon you notice that each beat is in sync with each droplet. The rhythm is perfect, comforting, and soothing.

Apply

Make a mental connection and apply how the dew-laden cherry blossom drips rhythmically into a glasslike inlet on the river's edge. Imagine how each drop falls in a steady, regular fashion and flows like your steady, flowing electrical system. Note that the beautiful vegetation around you represents your healthy heart. Listen to how the sounds of the gentle breeze blowing in the trees and the sound of the water droplets falling to the water's surface resemble your heart. You can hear the rhythm of your heart—constant, regular, and powerful.

Treat

View this exercise as a special treatment for yourself. You are deserving of this pleasurable and therapeutic time. The exercise is pleasurable, relaxing, and rejuvenating. This is not a chore or a task. Before long you will look forward to this work and feel like a runner who experiences a high from running.

Remember that this exercise, when performed correctly, is therapeutic and serves to decrease your heart rate, lower your blood pressure, and lower your vascular tone. The deeper and more relaxed you become, the more protective and effective is the therapy. Meditation and exercises such as B-R-E-A-T-H-E technique are therapeutic: they lower the levels of cardiotoxic hormones such as cortisol and adrenaline. This exercise increases heart-rate variability and low fluctuations in heart rate (low heart-rate variability) in patients who have been diagnosed with poor cardiovascular outcomes. Recall that guided imagery bolsters the immune system, lowers blood pressure and heart rate, and decreases anxiety.

Heal

When using the B-R-E-A-T-H-E technique, imagine the healing properties of relaxation. Your deep breathing helps you to train the nerves that connect the brain and the heart and has a calming and slowing effect on your heart rate. This exercise will reduce stress and make you feel better, which will enhance healing in your body. It will allow you to downshift so that your engine can cool and idle for a while. Imagine that the warm sun on your shoulders causes your blood vessels to dilate, further improving flow and thus healing your electrical system. Store the heart-healing metaphors in your memory so they can be quickly retrieved to help protect and heal your heart in a stressful situation.

End

As you end your B-R-E-A-T-H-E exercise, recall all of the heart-healing metaphors and summarize their significance and their relationship to your healing heart. Remember the perfectly flowing river, the beautiful cherry blossom, and the powerful waterfall. Recall the rhythmic dripping of the iridescent water droplets. As you end your exercise, you will become aware of your surroundings and feel energized. Your heart is strong, rhythmic, and unobstructed like the river.

6

Treating and Preventing Valve Disease

Mike Rossero, thirty-two, lives in a suburb of Philadelphia and has worked as a plumber for his father's firm, Rossero & Son Plumbing, since he was old enough to lug a wrench. He started accompanying his overly protective father when he was thirteen, and it seemed that every moment he wasn't in school as a teenager, he was helping his father to unclog stopped-up toilets, install sump pumps, repair leaky pipes, and clear sluggish drains.

For the first few years, he helped his father by carrying tools and acting as a parts runner, fetching parts from the truck. By the time the summer vacation between his junior and senior years in high school arrived, his entire life seemed to have been planned by his parents. He was the only son and thus expected to finish high school, spend two years at Delaware County Community College (DCCC), join his father's small plumbing business, find and marry a local girl (preferably of Italian heritage and who also attended St. Thomas Catholic Church), have a bunch of kids, and eventually buy a house on the same block as his parents. Mike, however, had a bigger dream.

Mike Rossero wanted to be an actor more than anything in the world. In grade school, his cherubic good looks and great singing voice had always gotten him cast in high school and college plays and musicals, and from the first time he'd run onstage—as one of the street urchins in *Oliver!*—he'd been hooked. To his parents' disappointment, throughout high school and during his two years at DCCC he had appeared in every play and musical he could manage. They thought it was a waste of time—a "pipe dream," they called it. His acting was a constant irritant and source of family arguments.

To his parents' further dismay, he hadn't married, didn't have a girlfriend (why bother, he reasoned, because one day, when he became famous, he'd marry a starlet), and didn't bowl or play softball with his old friends. By day—and most workdays were ten to twelve hours long—he wore his blue plumber's uniform with the No ORDINARY PLUMBER emblem on his cap and shirt, but by night (and on weekends) he lived his dream of working to be discovered and becoming a famous actor.

To catch a role in a community theater play or musical, Mike would generally show up at an open audition and succeed in gaining a part. A few days earlier, however, a woman named Beth from the Philadelphia Theater Company had left a message on his cell phone saying that the directors of the theater's upcoming production of *Hello, Dolly!* wanted him to audition for the role of Cornelius Hackl, one of the biggest roles in the show.

Mike bought the script and the music online and literally spent twenty-four hours a day for six straight days memorizing every line of the dialogue and the music. The role was his to lose, and he wasn't going to lose it.

He was so nervous about being late for the audition that he arrived at the theater two hours early, but because the auditions were open only to those reading and singing for a particular role, he wasn't allowed into the theater until thirty minutes before his call time. So he paced the streets, imagining the dance steps that would accompany the words to the song for the audition and becoming more nervous and anxious by the minute.

Finally, at exactly thirty minutes before his scheduled audition, the doorman allowed Mike into the theater, walked him to the front row, and directed him to have a seat until the accompanist and the codirectors returned from a short break. As he sat in the front row anxiously awaiting their return, he noticed a half-opened door off to the side of the stage and heard two male voices. He was able to make out the following fragments of conversation:

"I'm not sure he's . . ."

"I'm concerned about not enough musical . . ."

"Maybe we should think about someone else instead."

Hearing the negative bits of conversation behind the door, Mike immediately assumed that the comments were about him. He thought that the two men must be discussing his inexperience and shortcomings. His mind started racing and became filled with insecurity and self-doubt, and he began sweating and felt his heart race. Suddenly the men from behind the half-opened door appeared.

"Hi, Mike, glad you could make it," said one of the men, walking toward him and extending his hand.

"Mike," says the other man, "Bill and I are really pressed for time today, so if we could have you take the stage and give your music to the accompanist, we'll get started right away."

"Sure," says Mike.

As he stepped up onto the stage, he began to feel light-headed, and a distant memory flashed through his mind. Everything around him seemed to be graying out. His peripheral vision suddenly disappeared, as if he were a race horse wearing blinders. A wave of nausea rushed over him, and he was instantly drenched with sweat.

What was happening reminded Mike of the time in junior high school that he'd fainted after receiving a flu shot. He vividly recalled the school nurse hovering over him and saying something about a heart murmur. The light-headed feelings he was experiencing were surprisingly similar to that day back then.

In fact, Mike had the same combination of symptoms whenever he became stressed or nervous, and the same distant memory always haunted him. He often wondered if these frequent symptoms of feeling faint were related to a heart murmur that he'd never taken the time to investigate. From time to time he wondered if he should have his heart checked, but he always minimized its significance and rationalized that he was too young to have a heart problem.

Mike handed the music to the piano player and was about to take his place and wait for the opening notes of music when all of a sudden a deafening *baaammmmm* echoed through the theater, caused by the heavy metal backstage door slamming shut. Mike, startled by the noise, turned as white as a sheet, lost consciousness, fell, and struck his head on the hardwood floor.

One of the directors, trained in CPR, quickly grabbed the automated external defibrillator hanging on the wall of the theater, ripped open Mike's shirt, and attached the device to his chest.

Within moments the voice-activated machine identified a life-threatening arrhythmia and instructed the director to deliver a shock. The AED charged and sent a shock to Mike's heart, which caused his body to actually bounce off the hardwood floor.

Almost immediately, Mike sat bolt upright with blood trickling from a laceration above his left eyebrow and asked, "What happened?"

The Cardiac Cycle: Normally Functioning Heart Valves

Valvular heart disease affects the valves, the doorways of the heart's chambers that are responsible for directing blood from one chamber to another. The heart is like a house with four rooms, separated by four one-way doors: each chamber has one door that leads into it and one door that leads out of it.

Blood travels from the body and collects in the top right chamber of the heart, known as the right atrium, then flows down through a door to the second chamber, known as the right ventricle. From here the blood is propelled into the lungs and after collecting oxygen enters the top left side of the heart and the third chamber, known as the left atrium. This chamber is about the size of a plum. Once the left atrium is full, its door (think of a saloon door) opens and empties the contents into the fourth chamber, known as the left ventricle. The contraction of the left ventricle is what generates our pulse and our blood pressure. The left ventricle is the most important chamber of the heart because it is the main pump or engine for our circulatory system.

Once the left ventricle is full, it begins to squeeze the blood out another door, which leads to the brain and to the body. As the left ventricle contracts and propels the blood forward, it closes the door from the left atrium behind it. Thus, when the valves are working correctly, the blood moves forward from one room to the next through a series of one-way doorways in which one closes as the next one opens.

As the left ventricle contracts, the blood flows through the aortic valve into the aorta, which is a tube the diameter of a garden hose. The aorta connects the heart to the brain and the body. When all of the blood has gone through the door leading to the aorta from the left ventricle, the left ventricle relaxes and its door closes.

A diseased or defective heart valve is like a door that fails to either open or close fully. When a valve doesn't close completely and is left partially open, blood can leak backward. This backward flow through a valve is called *regurgitation*. When the hinges on the door become rusty, the valve fails to open completely and is called *stenosis*.

A Faulty Doorway:
When a Valve Fails to Open or
Close Correctly

Problems arise when the hinges of the valves become rusty and the valves fail to open or close appropriately. It is hard for the heart to pump blood through a door that's stuck or only partly open. Less blood is propelled through the door that connects to the brain and the body. Blood backs up into the lungs, causing various degrees of shortness of breath and congestive heart failure. When less blood is ejected to the brain and the body, people feel light-headed, dizzy, and easily fatigued.

Another common problem with the valves occurs when the saloonlike doors don't ever completely close, leading to a permanently leaky valve.

When the doors fail to open or close correctly, the flow of blood through the valve becomes turbulent, like a whitewater rapid coursing through boulders in a river. This high-velocity flow of blood creates the sound known as a heart murmur.

CARDIOLOGIST'S ANALYSIS
The Door Half Open

Mike made the first in a series of mistakes when he failed to listen to the concerns of the school nurse years ago. She correctly identified a murmur, the sound created by the turbulent blood flow through his blocked aortic valve. The hinges on this valve became progressively rustier, further depriving his brain and his body of blood and oxygen.

Mike was correct in his intuition that his symptoms of feeling tired and light-headed were related to his murmur. The severely blocked aortic valve made it difficult for his heart to pump blood forward to his brain and his body, especially when he was climbing stairs or running. "Burning the candle at both ends," as he tended to do, also took its toll.

When he showed up for the rehearsal, Mike was in bad shape: sleep-deprived, dehydrated, and stressed, and now with the additional stress of stage fright. These are all known causes of fainting, which is even more likely when coupled with a blocked aortic valve.

The final trigger of Mike's fainting episode was a loud noise caused by the slamming of a heavy metal door backstage. This sudden noise literally almost scared him to death. Mike's stress response was stimulated, causing a massive release of stress hormones, which made his heart muscle irritable and triggered a nearly fatal arrhythmia. Acting quickly, the director saved Mike's life by shocking him back into a stable cardiac rhythm.

When Your Heart Murmurs, Listen

Aortic valve stenosis arises when the hinges on the door that connects the main pumping chamber to the brain and the body become rusty. The stress is put on the main pumping chamber, or aorta, because it has to generate tremendous force to exit the heart through a partly blocked door. As the heart squeezes with all its might, it creates a high-velocity flow through the valve—like putting your thumb over the end of a garden hose and making the water flow faster and more turbulently. This fast-flowing, turbulent flow creates the sound known as a heart murmur. Mike's nurse in junior high school had heard this murmur years ago. Over time, Mike's valve had progressively narrowed, and he developed typical symptoms. The three most common are the following:

1. Difficulty breathing due to a backup of blood into the lungs
2. Dizziness due to less blood traveling to the brain
3. Chest pain due to inadequate blood flow to the thickened heart muscle

The Causes of Aortic Stenosis

Mike had a congenital variety of aortic stenosis known as congenital bicuspid aortic stenosis. Normally the aortic valve has three saloonlike doorways but someone with this form of aortic stenosis is born with only two, which makes the valve prone to leaking and blockage.

Following is a list of all the causes of aortic stenosis:

- *Congenital aortic stenosis*   Some people are born with a narrow aortic valve. The most common form of congenital aortic stenosis is the type that our patient has: bicuspid aortic stenosis. Mike's aortic valve has only two flaps instead of three. If you've been diagnosed with congenital aortic valve stenosis, you should see your doctor regularly, watching for the signs and symptoms previously mentioned.

- *Calcium buildup on the valve*   As we age, the hinges on our heart valves become calcified. Over time the calcification can lead to a severely blocked aortic valve. Calcification narrows the aortic valve, and *calcific aortic stenosis* is the most common form of aortic stenosis. Heart valves themselves (rather than just their hinges) can also accumulate deposits of calcium. This is called *aortic valve calcification,* and as blood flows through the aortic valve, the calcium deposits accumulate on the valve's leaflets. High cholesterol contributes to degenerative changes in the aortic valve. Unlike bicuspid aortic stenosis, which Mike has, patients with calcific aortic stenosis tend to experience symptoms later in life—usually in their sixties and seventies.

- *Rheumatic valvulitis*   Rheumatic heart disease is the most common cause of aortic stenosis worldwide, but it is extremely unusual in the United States. That's because it's a complication of untreated strep throat. It used to be common in our country, but with the advent and availability of penicillin, we have almost eradicated the disease. Over time, patients with rheumatic fever develop antibodies that attack the aortic valve, causing it to become inflamed and thickened. Scar tissue then develops, causing the valve to become blocked.

- *Radiation*   Some patients who receive radiation for cancer develop a thickening of their aortic valve as a side effect. Radiation therapy is believed to weaken the aortic valve, making it vulnerable to calcification and stenosis.

- *Medication side effect*   In rare cases, medications for migraine headaches that contain ergotamine can lead to aortic stenosis.

Aortic valve stenosis often isn't preventable. If you have a murmur, you should consult your doctor to make sure that you are monitored appropriately. Mike was born with aortic stenosis, and although the course of his disease would not have changed, he could have been prepared for surgery over time and have scheduled surgery on an elective rather than an emergency basis. If you have a heart murmur, make sure you consult a physician.

Diagnosing Valve Disease

The odds are that at some point in your life you've had a physical exam in which a health-care provider listened to your heart with a stethoscope.

If a murmur is discovered, as in Mike's case, the nurse or the doctor will mention it to you and will typically recommend or arrange further testing to determine the cause. The actual murmur is a sound created by the turbulent flow through the valve, like the roar of a whitewater rapid through boulders in a river.

The following diagnostic tests are done for a heart murmur:

- *Electrocardiogram (ECG)*   This is a test of the heart's electrical system. It can give your doctor clues about your heart's chamber sizes and the thickness of your heart muscle—typical changes and findings caused by aortic stenosis.

- *Chest X-ray* A chest X-ray will help your doctor to determine if your heart is enlarged or if there is any fluid buildup in your lungs; the cause of shortness of breath from aortic stenosis. Calcium and a dilated aorta can also be seen on a regular chest X-ray.

- *Echocardiogram* This is an ultrasound of your heart and will typically give your doctor the most important information about the severity of your valve condition. In general, doctors report a continuum of disease, ranging from mild to moderate to severe. When Mike arrived at the emergency room, an echocardiogram revealed severe aortic stenosis. Other conditions, such as thickened heart muscle and enlarged heart chambers, were also seen.

- *Cardiac catheterization* This is an invasive procedure that is usually recommended before an aortic valve replacement. In addition to carefully evaluating the aortic valve, your cardiologist will evaluate your coronary arteries. The cardiologist will access your heart through a vein and an artery located in your leg or your arm. Next your doctor will thread a thin tube through your heart, using a specially designed device known as a catheter. A special liquid known as contrast will then be injected through the arteries, mimicking the flow of blood through them. This special substance is visible under X-ray and allows the cardiologist to see any blockages. Other important information obtained during this procedure includes how much blood your heart pumps in liters and minutes, which is known as your cardiac output. At the conclusion of this procedure, your doctor will have all the pieces of the puzzle to repair your heart parts.

The Complications of Valve Disease

If not carefully monitored, patients with aortic stenosis can develop symptoms that can be potentially life-threatening. As the valve narrows and becomes progressively blocked, congestive heart failure, angina, and even sudden death can occur from strain on the heart. Aortic stenosis also increases the risk of infection, because the lining or surface of the valve is roughed up and vulnerable to infection.

Until 2007 doctors recommended taking antibiotics before procedures (such as dental work) that increased the risk of bacteria getting into your blood. However, we found that few patients actually required antibiotics, which led to new recommendations. Your doctor will tell you if antibiotics are necessary for you before such a procedure.

The Timing of Surgery

Aortic stenosis is a progressive disease. In some cases it progresses slowly and doesn't require surgical therapy. Sometimes, however, it progresses rapidly and goes from mild to severe. There is no way of truly knowing the rate of progression; if you have aortic stenosis, you should be monitored by a cardiologist.

Medications

Recent research suggests that a class of cholesterol-lowering medications known as statins may prevent aortic valve stenosis or slow its progression in some patients with blood cholesterol abnormalities.

If you have either a bicuspid aortic valve or various degrees of aortic stenosis, ask your doctor if you are a candidate for a statin drug. If you have aortic stenosis, antibiotics for preventing endocarditis are no longer required, but your cardiologist should discuss this with you.

Surgery

The two most frequently performed surgical fixes for valve disease include:

- *Aortic valve replacement* This is the most conventional and effective way to treat severe aortic stenosis. There are a number of different types of valves, which are either bioprosthetic (pig, cow, or human) or mechanical. There are a number of considerations to be addressed when choosing the type of valve replacement. This decision is best made by the patient, the cardiologist, and the surgeon. Some issues that help to determine the type of valve are age, risk of bleeding, and lifestyle. The type of valve should be discussed with you and your doctors.

- *Balloon valvuloplasty* This procedure is used when the patient is not a candidate for aortic valve replacement. A thin guide wire is passed through the thickened valve. A thin cylindrical balloon is passed over the wire and positioned at the level of the blocked valve. The balloon is then inflated, and the valve is cracked open. Aortic valve balloon valvuloplasty is used most often in infants and children and very rarely in adults.

Our Patient

Mike, the aspiring actor, experienced an episode of sudden death. He was rapidly resuscitated, and 911 was called. Paramedics brought Mike to the hospital, where an emergency room doctor heard a murmur and ordered an echocardiogram. This clinched the diagnosis of severe aortic stenosis.

The echocardiogram also gave clues to the cause of the blocked valve. It appeared that Mike was born with an abnormal valve known as a bicuspid aortic valve. This type of abnormal aortic valve is the second most common cause of aortic stenosis in the United States. Although his murmur had been recognized in grade school, he had gone through life not knowing of his serious heart condition. For many people with this form of aortic stenosis, the diagnosis is unknown until they develop symptoms of shortness of breath, dizziness, or chest pain. Some patients with this condition have an infection on the valve, which is a common complication.

Mike subsequently underwent successful aortic valve surgery and was recovering nicely when his hospital stay took one final unexpected turn. Just two days after his surgery, an ICU nurse noticed a number of skipped beats (known as PVCs) on his heart monitor and called the cardiologist for further review. These skipped beats revealed yet another clue to the cause of Mike's fainting episode. Although it seemed logical that stress from performance anxiety and dehydration along with a severely blocked aortic valve explained his fainting episode, another explanation involved the suddenly slamming door, which seemed to trigger Mike's fainting episode and nearly fatal heart rhythm. Mike was nearly scared to death. Further analysis of Mike's electrical cardiac system revealed a diagnosis known as "long-QT syndrome." In this disorder, loud noises have been reported to precipitate sudden cardiac death due to fatal arrhythmias. In one study, patients with a congenital form of aortic stenosis were found to be more likely to have this electrical abnormality and thus to be sensitive to sudden loud noises that potentially lead to lethal arrhythmias.

To treat this problem, Mike had an additional procedure known as a pacemaker ICD (implantable cardioverter defibrillator), which prevented any further abnormal heart rhythms.

Mike has been asymptomatic since his heart surgery and attributes his good health to practicing his B-R-E-A-T-H-E technique. He has stopped working as a plumber, works regularly as an actor in film and onstage, and teaches an acting workshop that emphasizes fighting stage fright.

B-R-E-A-T-H-E

The Boulders Exercise

This exercise should be done by patients with aortic stenosis or those who have had aortic valve surgery.

Begin

Begin your exercise in your warm, cozy, and familiar place. Wear loose-fitting clothing and settle comfortably in your favorite chair or sofa. Always start your exercise by listening to the conversation. Remember that your heart and your brain are connected and in constant communication. Listen to your heart.

Take a deep breath in through your nose and let it out through your mouth. Count s-l-o-w-l-y to seven. Notice that when you take in a deep breath, your heart rate slightly increases, and as you exhale, your heart rate decreases. Take a few more breaths and notice this trend: in, your heart rate increases; out, your heart rate decreases. The more you practice, the better you will get at hearing your heartbeat. This is excellent proof that you are participating in the conversation.

As you begin, focus on your heart and clear your mind of any other thoughts. Liken this exercise to working out different muscles in the gym. Instead of working your back, your shoulders, or your biceps, look at this exercise as exercising and developing your heart-brain connection.

Relax

Remember that the relaxation response is a state of deep relaxation that is the opposite of the fight-or-flight response. You can reach this state by deep breathing. It is comfortable, soothing, and nurturing for your heart. Breathing in and out causes changes in the heart rate. When you take a deep breath in, you are activating the sympathetic nervous system, which causes your heart rate to speed up. When you exhale, count to seven, like the number of letters in B-R-E-A-T-H-E. This extended exhalation activates the parasympathetic nervous system and slows the heart rate by sending signals from your brain to your heart on a highway called the vagus nerve. This fluctuation or variability of the heart rate is good for the heart.

Envision

Imagine sitting at the foot of a river. As you gaze down the majestic river, you notice two enormous boulders that have tumbled down the mountain and come to rest next to each other in the middle of the river. You marvel at the size of the rocks and imagine their excessive weight.

The two massive stones sitting side by side have a small space between them, which generates a powerful whitewater rapid. The turbulent flow creates a high-pitched roar that can be heard in the deep forest miles away.

You turn your head gently to the left and notice the powerful waterfall. You watch as the waterfall builds momentum and drives the river forward, pushing the massive stones apart. The massive boulders, once an impediment to the flowing river, are pushed gently end over end, finally settling on the shore. The roar of the transient whitewater rapid is gone.

You hear only the soft, gentle bubbling and trickling of the unimpeded river and the distant roar of the waterfall.

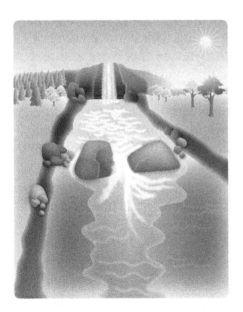 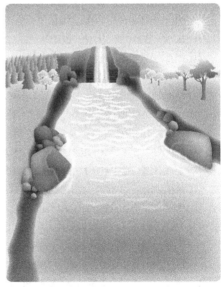

Apply

Apply how the two massive boulders are like your heart valve. Initially you observe how they are perfectly positioned in the middle of the majestic river, sitting side by side with only a small space between them. Note how they impede the forward flow of the river and how the small space between them creates a turbulent jetty or rapid. Apply how the powerful river is like your powerful heart and marvel as the flowing river gathers momentum from the power of the waterfall and then pushes the boulders to the shore of the river, effortlessly clearing its path and flow. Focus on this image and apply how this is like the forward flow across your perfectly functioning heart valve. It opens and closes perfectly, allowing forward flow to your body parts just as the freely flowing river provides its banks with lush vegetation.

Treat

View this exercise as a special treatment for yourself. You are deserving of this pleasurable and therapeutic time. The exercise is pleasurable, relaxing, and rejuvenating. This is not a chore or a task. Before long you will look forward to this work and feel like a runner who experiences a high from running.

Remember that this exercise, when performed correctly, is therapeutic and serves to decrease your heart rate, lower your blood pressure, and lower your vascular tone. The deeper and more relaxed you become, the more protective and effective is the therapy. Meditation and exercises such as B-R-E-A-T-H-E technique are therapeutic: they lower the levels of cardio-toxic hormones such as cortisol and adrenaline. This exercise increases heart-rate variability and low fluctuations in heart rate (low heart-rate variability) in patients who have been diagnosed with poor cardiovascular outcomes. Recall that guided imagery bolsters the immune system, lowers blood pressure and heart rate, and decreases anxiety.

Heal

When using the B-R-E-A-T-H-E technique, imagine the healing properties of relaxation. Your deep breathing helps you to train the nerves that connect the brain and the heart and has a calming and slowing effect on your heart rate. This exercise will reduce stress and make you feel better, which will enhance healing in your body. It will allow you to downshift so that your engine can cool and idle for a while. Imagine that the warm sun on your shoulders causes your blood vessels to dilate, further improving flow and thus healing your electrical system. Store the heart-healing metaphors in your memory so they can be quickly retrieved to help protect and heal your heart in a stressful situation.

End

As you end your B-R-E-A-T-H-E exercise, recall all of the heart-healing metaphors and summarize their significance and their relationship to your healing heart. Remember the perfectly flowing river, the powerful waterfall, and the large granite boulders. Recall the powerful waterfall and the flowing river as it gently pushes the boulders to shore. As you end your exercise, you will become aware of your surroundings and feel energized. Your heart is strong, rhythmic, and unobstructed like the river.

7

B-R-E-A-T-H-E for Everyone

Bill and Millie Dahlberg were a beautiful couple. They began dating when they were in high school, married immediately upon Bill's return to the United States after a three-year hitch in the army, and began a wonderful life together.

Bill ran the family hardware and lumber business that had been handed down to him by his father, and he built it from fewer than ten employees to more than three hundred. Millie was a magazine editor who also loved writing poetry and volunteering in church.

By the time they became my patients, they had been married sixty years and had three children, nine grandchildren, and a large wave of great-grandchildren that had just begun arriving.

Millie had retired, but at age eighty-two, Bill still spent four days a week overseeing the business, which he ran jointly with his son and his grandson.

Bill and Millie did everything together and traveled frequently. When they weren't jaunting off on a cruise or to some exotic locale, they were busy with Little League, junior high, and high school athletic contests—and, in their words, "spoiling the grandchildren and the great-grandchildren."

I was honored to have them as my patients. I enjoyed hearing stories of their recent travels as well as tales of their grandchildren and great-grandchildren's escapades and accomplishments.

One Christmas morning, while getting the house ready for the huge family celebration, Bill and his son, Joe, went outside to move a load of firewood from the backyard woodpile into the living room and the family room.

As Bill was stacking the last log onto the wheelbarrow, he suddenly told Joe that he felt as if a shade had been pulled down over his eyes, obscuring his vision. At this point he sat down on a tree stump, slumped over, and lost consciousness. Joe called for help and started CPR, but despite his and the paramedics' best efforts, Bill never regained consciousness. He passed away.

I continued to see and care for Millie after Bill's death, and, except for mildly elevated cholesterol, she remained the picture of health. However, almost a year after Bill's death, something started happening with clockwork precision.

Each November I would see Mille for her annual checkup and she would be fine, but a few weeks later she'd develop a fever, chills, a cough that produced phlegm, and rapid heart palpitations, which required hospitalization and treatment with intravenous antibiotics for her pneumonia and potent anti-arrhythmic medications for her heart rhythm.

After her third annual December admission to the hospital, I asked if she thought there might be a connection between her annual illness and the anniversary of Bill's death. At first she vigorously denied any connection, but after a few minutes of discussion she admitted to having feelings of anxiety and overwhelming feelings of residual grief. She said that the worst part was the entire family tiptoeing around the subject and purposely avoiding talking about Bill around Christmas because they thought it would upset her. Unfortunately, all the repression fueled her anxieties even more, which stressed her immune system and made her vulnerable to recurrent pneumonia.

The solution was the creation of a new family tradition. Early each Christmas morning, Millie would go by herself to the lake where she and Bill had gone on daily walks. She would sit at the edge of the lake and inhale the fresh, clean air and practice her B-R-E-A-T-H-E technique. Later, at the start of Christmas dinner, each person would make a toast to Bill about a pleasant memory of his or her late father, grandfather, or great-grandfather. Miraculously, Millie breathed comfortably for the next eight Decembers and remained pneumonia-free.

White-Coat Hypertension

The first time I saw my new patient, Tom Heath, his blood pressure was elevated. He quickly dismissed it by saying, "Oh, that always happens when I go to a doctor," adding, "I have white-coat hypertension."

When I asked why he felt compelled to see a cardiologist if he was so healthy, he told me that his family has a history of heart disease, so he wanted a thorough checkup. My intuition told me that Tom's outward appearance was very different from what was going on inside him.

Tom is a partner in a huge law firm with a bunch of names in the firm's title (his is one of them). His specialty is litigation, and he prides himself on loving his work, thriving, and remaining cool under pressure.

Intrigued by the disparity between Tom's perception of being cool under pressure and his consistently high blood-pressure recordings, I asked how he was able to achieve his sense of calm in pressure-cooker situations. He told me that he feels so relaxed because he is committed to life-work balance and takes a two-week vacation every three months. I applauded him for recognizing how stressful his job was and for balancing his life by taking time off.

During our third meeting in three months, I took his blood pressure and again recorded a reading of 190/98. I explained to him that this was more than white-coat hypertension and that his blood pressure would have to be treated. However, his blood pressure was incredibly difficult to control. Even after multiple medications, a cutback in alcohol consumption, and regular exercise, his blood pressure remained elevated. Finally, to make sure that there wasn't another cause for his refractory hypertension, I asked him how he relaxed when he took time off.

Tom proudly told me about his beautiful condo on the shores of Kauai, his private beach, and his favorite hammock. Then he told me about his relaxation ritual. First he'd get comfortable in his hammock and check his BlackBerry for any recent messages. He explained that he loved work so much that he had to stay in the loop *just a little* while on vacation. Then he'd check in with his secretary to make sure that all was well and that the fort was secure in his absence. Then he'd take a much-needed nap.

I asked him if he saw anything stressful about his ritual, and his response was, "Absolutely not, Doc, that's my secret of why I'm so cool under pressure."

I told him that leaving work at work would probably help him to truly relax. Then I explained the importance of the heart-brain connection; that when we are stressed, our stress hormones lead to elevated blood pressure; and that his constant worry about his firm was stimulating his stress response and contributing to his elevated blood pressure.

I explained the importance of understanding that listening to the heart-brain conversation and learning to relax required concentration and focus. Even though Tom was taking time off work, lounging in a hammock, and catching up on sleep, this isn't as effective as focused and conscious relaxation. After Tom learned the B-R-E-A-T-H-E technique, his blood pressure fell ten points. Before long, we had figured out the successful remedy. He left his BlackBerry at home while on vacation, practiced B-R-E-A-T-H-E daily, exercised, avoided salt in his diet, and took one 12.5-milligram tablet of hydrochlorothiazide daily. Before long, we were getting nearly normal blood-pressure readings of 125/82, even with his white-coat hypertension.

CARDIOLOGIST'S ANALYSIS
The Perils of Repressed Anxiety

Although otherwise completely healthy, Millie and Tom were both stricken by stress-related illnesses. Tom's repression of his job stress and Millie's repression of her feelings of loss were harmful to the health of both individuals.

Tom repressed his anxiety about the tremendous pressures and responsibilities of running a high-profile law firm, and it manifested in high blood pressure. For Millie, the anniversary of her husband's death created tremendous unacknowledged anxiety and stress. Without fail, the emotional storm weakened her immune system, making her vulnerable to infection, until on Christmas Day each year she was admitted to the hospital with full-blown pneumonia and rapid palpitations. The low oxygen levels caused by the pneumonia and the elevated adrenaline levels from her grief-related anxiety caused her heart to go into an arrhythmia known as paroxysmal supra-ventricular tachycardia (PSVT).

Both individuals had had reminders of the heart-brain conversation but had chosen to ignore them. Tom felt sweaty before having to perform in the courtroom, and Millie felt a queasy feeling in her stomach. In both cases, lowering their stress levels greatly helped to decrease their output of stress hormones, which was contributing to their conditions. Once the triggers were accurately identified, the B-R-E-A-T-H-E technique helped them both to battle stress and overcome the pattern of their conditions. Now they're both aware of the triggers and have developed reliable and effective stress management strategies with the help of B-R-E-A-T-H-E.

Stress at Work

If you are like most people, you are part of the workforce and are required to work for a living to provide food and shelter for yourself and perhaps a family as well. In a large study of factory workers in Britain, people who reported stress and high anxiety at work were 67 percent more likely to develop heart disease over a twelve-year period than those who said they felt comfortable and calm in the workplace. Those who were under fifty and said that their work was stressful were nearly 70 percent more likely to develop heart disease than those who were under fifty and reported being stress-free.

In addition to eating poorly and exercising less, those who were stressed also showed abnormal blood cholesterol, blood sugar, and insulin levels. Specifically, they were less likely to eat sufficient amounts of fruit and vegetables and were less likely to exercise, so their lifestyle definitely contributed to the development of heart disease. If you are feeling stressed at work and your intuition tells you that it's not good for you, your intuition is probably right.

Learn to Leave Work at Work

According to a recent report, some workers at an Internet company in Seattle were frustrated with their counterparts in Ireland because at five o'clock in the afternoon, Dublin time (which is nine in the morning, Seattle time), Irish workers left their cubicles and went to the local pub to lift a pint with their friends. Nevertheless, the Irish office was just as effective as the Seattle office in terms of productivity. The focus was on work until five and then elsewhere thereafter. Americans could stand to learn a thing or two from this work mentality; it would lead to a healthier and more productive workplace.

Many of us are addicted to work or are afraid to leave it, no matter how stressful it might be. We need to understand the importance of not only taking time off from work and enjoying regular vacations but also learning to incorporate relaxation into our everyday routine.

Relaxation: It's Harder Than You Think

It should be pretty clear by now that the premise of this book is that stress is incontrovertibly bad for your heart and that relaxation is extraordinarily beneficial—as the data clearly show. Yet Americans, for some reason, have trouble letting go and learning to relax. Living in our fast-paced world filled with deadlines, work pressures, relationship needs, and family and friend obligations, we are all keenly aware of the need to relax. Unfortunately, most of us rarely take the time to do so.

A recent study that analyzed cultural work ethics showed that Europeans take three more weeks of vacation a year than age-matched Americans do. The travel agency Expedia.com recently completed its Vacation Deprivation Survey, which showed that Americans receive the fewest vacation days (fourteen) per year, compared to seventeen days in Australia, nineteen days in Canada, twenty-four days in Britain, twenty-seven days in Germany, and thirty-nine days in France.

A survey published in the *Financial Post*, entitled "Too Busy to Take a Vacation," showed that once we finally do break away from work—which requires actually turning off the cell phone, putting away the BlackBerry, and putting on a floral shirt and a pair of flip-flops—we have trouble relaxing.

According to the Hudson Group in New York City, more than 50 percent of U.S. workers fail to take all their vacation days, and 15 percent give up their vacation entirely. Even though we know it's good for us to take a breather, most of us don't. The current economy and workplace, plagued with layoffs and cutbacks, puts an employee in a very difficult situation. Budget cuts and layoffs mean more work for fewer people, which means that working people deserve and need their vacation time even more than usual.

Yet how can people take time off when they have too much work and are worried about their job security? Moreover, the irrational guilt some of us feel during our absence, thinking that we are overburdening our colleagues, makes it impossible to relax. All that worry is exhausting, and by the time we return to work, we are ready for a real vacation. In fact, in a nationwide survey of 2,082 workers done by the Rasmussen Group, 21 percent reported returning to work feeling more stressed than when they left.

A vacation should be relaxing and pleasurable and should reenergize and rejuvenate you. If you do it right and refill your energy meter, the time away might even help you to bring fresh ideas to the table. Also, when you plan a vacation in advance, you will look organized and professional to, as well as considerate of, your colleagues and senior leadership, which will help rather than harm your job security.

If we accept that we are all faced with pressures at work and that stress that is ignored can be harmful to our health, then we can agree that we need to learn a simple relaxation technique to use in the daily workplace. The following messages are clear:

- We all have stress at work, and we need to learn how to manage it.
- We should take our well-deserved and much-needed vacation time; we can't afford not to!
- We need to learn to leave work at work.

In addition, we all need to develop coping skills like the B-R-E-A-T-H-E technique to help us endure daily challenges and manage stress in the workplace. Even if you love your job, you owe it to yourself to learn this stress-relieving technique.

Red Flags

When we have multiple obligations and more responsibilities than usual—project deadlines, mortgage payments, weddings and birthdays all falling within the same week—we might not consider ourselves stressed. However, if we were aware of all the activity inside our bodies that has been caused by all the added pressure, most of us would be surprised. Although we might not feel stressed, a hormonal storm can be brewing within. In such situations, many of us often tend to minimize how hectic life can be, and we become even more neglectful of how this negatively affects our body.

Stress can have a negative impact on all of us, healthy or not. No matter how low your cholesterol is or how soon you finished your last ten-kilometer run, stress is part of our lives and can be harmful if ignored. Whether you are dealing with the anniversary of a traumatic event, a "white-coat" syndrome, work stress, or a difficult relationship, learning to manage stress is in your best interest, and the B-R-E-A-T-H-E technique can really help.

Recent studies in neuroscience suggest that all of us possess the ability to effectively manage stress; this is true even if you're the kind of person who typically sees the glass as half empty. We're all wired the same way and have the same "software" that allows us to consciously choose how to respond to stress. We can choose to respond destructively, by acting out with tantrums and emotional outbursts, or we can respond constructively, with calm, cool, and appropriate behavior. The B-R-E-A-T-H-E technique will help you to develop your brain to make a constructive response more probable.

What do you have to lose, other than a few points on your blood pressure and heart rate? B-R-E-A-T-H-E is applicable and helpful for everyone. It's a simple relaxation tool that will help you to feel great, focus, concentrate, and perform at your best.

The following exercise is designed to help anyone who accepts the notion that stress exists in all our lives and that it is important to learn ways to effectively manage it.

For best results, use the B-R-E-A-T-H-E technique as part of your daily routine and consider it as important as diet and exercise. It will improve your overall health as well as your outlook on life.

B-R-E-A-T-H-E
A General Exercise

By virtue of being human, we all have stress, and the vast majority of us have an asymptomatic form of heart disease. Studies show that the earliest marker for atherosclerosis, known as the fatty streak, is found in almost every three-year-old child in North America. Fatty streaks are caused by deposition of cholesterol in the walls of the arteries. Luckily, though the disease is likely to be brewing in most of us, not all will suffer from cardiac events. Those at greatest risk have one or more of the traditional risk factors, which include high blood pressure, high cholesterol, diabetes, smoking, and a family history of premature coronary artery disease. It is crucial then to treat modifiable risk factors to decrease the risk of a cardiac event. Stress is an example of a modifiable risk factor much like high cholesterol, high blood pressure, diabetes, and smoking. Therefore, all of us stand to benefit greatly by learning how to manage stress and by practicing the B-R-E-A-T-H-E technique.

This exercise is designed for people who have no history of heart disease but who at times feel stressed—whether it's the pressure to deliver a project on time or a speech at the local union hall. This exercise will be pleasurable and relaxing. If practiced regularly, it will help you to deal with stress in a pinch.

Concentrate on the following heart-healing metaphors:

- The waterfall is your powerful heart pump.
- The river is your smooth, unobstructed coronary arteries.
- The water droplets are your cardiac electrical system.
- The tree root represents your heart valves.

Begin

Begin your exercise in your warm, cozy, and familiar place. Wear loose-fitting clothing and settle comfortably in your favorite chair or sofa. Always start your exercise by listening to the conversation. Remember that your heart and your brain are connected and in constant communication. Listen to your heart.

Take a deep breath in through your nose and let it out through your mouth. Count s-l-o-w-l-y to seven. Notice that when you take in a deep breath, your heart rate slightly increases, and as you exhale, your heart rate decreases. Take a few more breaths and notice this trend: in, your heart rate increases; out, your heart rate decreases. The more you practice, the better you will get at hearing your heartbeat. This is excellent proof that you are participating in the conversation.

As you begin, focus on your heart and clear your mind of any other thoughts. Liken this exercise to working out different muscles in the gym. Instead of working your back, your shoulders, or your biceps, look at this exercise as exercising and developing your heart-brain connection.

Relax

Remember that the relaxation response is a state of deep relaxation that is the opposite of the fight-or-flight response. You can reach this state by deep breathing. It is comfortable, soothing, and nurturing for your heart. Breathing in and out causes changes in the heart rate. When you take a deep breath in, you are activating the sympathetic nervous system, which causes your heart rate to speed up. When you exhale, count to seven, like the number of letters in B-R-E-A-T-H-E. This extended exhalation activates the parasympathetic nervous system and slows the heart rate by sending signals from your brain to your heart on a highway called the vagus nerve. This fluctuation or variability of the heart rate is good for the heart.

Walk the path of relaxation and flow (see chapter 4). The sights and sounds are soothing, and as you take each step you become more conscious of your breathing. Your breathing and walking are in sync, and with each step you become more and more relaxed. You recognize this path and associate it with feelings of warmth, contentment, and peace, and you feel as though you've walked this path thousands of times before. The soft dust on your feet, the warm sun on your shoulders, and the fresh, clean, crisp air make you feel comfortable, secure, and relaxed. Each step is familiar, comforting, and soothing.

Envision

At the end of the path, an inviting bright light created by the sun's reflection on the river welcomes you to the river's edge, where you sit comfortably, relaxed and ready to start your heart-healing exercise. Imagine sitting at the foot of the river; notice the roar of the powerful waterfall. Imagine how it resembles your strong, healthy heart pump. Imagine how your powerful heart pump collects oxygenated blood from the lungs and then forcefully contracts, providing the body with blood. Imagine how this is like the waterfall, which collects water from the local rivulets, streams, and creeks and then provides a downstream flow to vegetation and wildlife. Think of how your heart muscle and pump are working perfectly.

See how the waterfall generates the current and constant unobstructed flow down the river, like the perfect flow of blood through your three perfect, smoothly lined coronary arteries. Imagine how the river carries nutrients to the local wildlife and vegetation, as your coronary arteries provide oxygen to nourish the healthy cardiac tissues. Think of how your coronary arteries are perfect and provide unobstructed flow to your heart muscle.

Over your left shoulder you notice a hanging branch from a nearby oak tree, which has collected the mist created by the powerful waterfall. You watch as the mist collects, slides down to the tip of the branch, and drips rhythmically into the glasslike inlet at the river's edge. As you watch each perfect droplet form and fall in a predictable and rhythmic fashion, you hear your heart as it beats in sync with each droplet. Imagine how this clocklike dripping from the branch is like the natural pacemaker and electrical system in your healthy heart. Think of how the flow of electricity in your heart is perfect.

As you look down at the riverbank, you notice a small twig-like root that protrudes into the river. You notice a to-and-fro motion that is determined by the current of the river. The motion of the root goes forward with the current, then back to idle position as the current slows, reminding you of the opening and

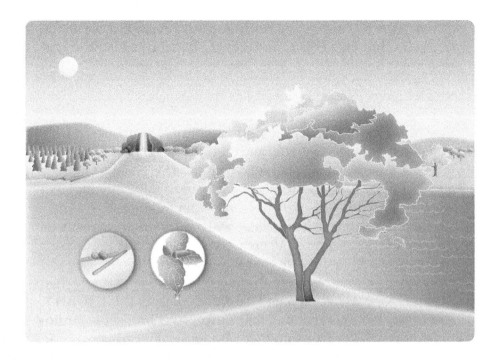

closing of your heart valves. Think of how the valves in your heart are opening and closing perfectly.

Apply

Make a mental connection and apply how the wide, smooth path is like your blood vessels. Imagine how the waterfall is like your strong heart pump. The freely flowing river represents your coronary arteries, the tree root that sways forward with the current then back to idle position is like your heart valves, and the water droplets that fall rhythmically into the glasslike inlet represent your perfectly flowing electrical system. You imagine how the heart muscle and pump, coronary arteries, valves, and electrical system are all working together perfectly. Apply how the waterfall, which powers the river, provides nutrients for the lush vegetation and is like your heart, which nourishes your healthy body.

Listen to the sounds around you: the gentle breeze blowing in the trees, the chirping of birds, and the sound of the distant waterfall resemble your heart—constant, rhythmic, and powerful.

Treat

View this exercise as a special treatment for yourself. You are deserving of this pleasurable and therapeutic time. The exercise is pleasurable, relaxing, and rejuvenating. This is not a chore or a task. Before long you will look forward to this work and feel like a runner who experiences a high from running.

Remember that this exercise, when performed correctly, is therapeutic and serves to decrease your heart rate, lower your blood pressure, and lower your vascular tone. The deeper and more relaxed you become, the more protective and effective is the therapy. Meditation and exercises such as B-R-E-A-T-H-E technique are therapeutic: they lower the levels of cardio-toxic hormones such as cortisol and adrenaline. This exercise increases heart-rate variability and low fluctuations in heart rate (low heart-rate variability) in patients who have been diagnosed with poor cardiovascular outcomes. Recall that guided imagery bolsters the immune system, lowers blood pressure and heart rate, and decreases anxiety.

Heal

When using the B-R-E-A-T-H-E technique, imagine the healing properties of relaxation. Your deep breathing helps you to train the nerves that connect the brain and the heart and has a calming and slowing effect on your heart rate. This exercise will reduce stress and make you feel better, which will enhance healing in your body. It will allow you to downshift so that your engine can cool and idle for a while. Imagine that the warm sun on your shoulders causes your blood vessels to dilate, further improving flow and thus healing your electrical system. Store the heart-healing metaphors in your memory so they can be quickly retrieved to help protect and heal your heart in a stressful situation.

End

As you end your B-R-E-A-T-H-E exercise, recall all of the heart-healing metaphors and summarize their significance and their relationship to your healing heart. Remember the powerful waterfall, the perfectly flowing river, the tree root, and the water droplets and imagine how they represent your heart pump, coronary arteries, heart valves, and electrical system respectively. As you end your exercise, you will become aware of your surroundings and feel energized. Your heart is strong, rhythmic, and unobstructed like the freely flowing river.

8

Fast Help: Stressed Out and Overloaded

You can use the B-R-E-A-T-H-E technique when you're up to your ears with stress, when you feel overwhelmed and there's seemingly no way out. In order to understand how the B-R-E-A-T-H-E technique applies in this situation, the interconnectedness of the heart, the mind, and the brain must be crystal clear.

The stress response involves a chain reaction that affects all of one's body and psyche, but nothing more than the brain, the mind, and the heart. (The brain and the heart are parts of our anatomy, and the mind is what gives us conscience, personality, thought process, and individual identity.) You'll see how each is activated in a predictable and repetitious sequence. Besides learning the sequence of events that occurs when we become stressed, you'll learn how the B-R-E-A-T-H-E technique can be used at a specific point in the cycle to stop stress in its tracks.

You'll learn how practicing the B-R-E-A-T-H-E technique can train the neural fibers that help you to develop an effective coping strategy, so that you can call on them in a pinch when your engine is running hot. (It's a bit like exercising your arm muscles to keep them in shape so that when you need to lift something heavy, you can.) It will improve your emotional vitality, calm and cool your engine, and ultimately protect your heart—even in the most stressful situations.

The History and Evolution of Stress

Our reaction to stress begins with a trigger, or fear stimulus, which sets off a chain reaction. The classic example involves the proverbial caveman with the saber-toothed tiger. Just the sight of the ferocious animal led to a flooding of the stress hormones adrenaline and cortisol. This shifted the caveman's organs into overdrive, which leads to one of three possible responses: fight, flight, or freeze. Originally this response protected us from danger and allowed us to procreate.

The consistent cascade of physiological changes that occurs when we're exposed to danger still protects us today. Long after the extinction of the saber-toothed tiger, the human response to a life-threatening situation—known as *the stress response*—has remained virtually unchanged.

Everything—the trigger, the release of hormones, the internal physiology, and the bodily response to the potential damage to the delicate cardiac tissue—is exactly the same.

Since the time of the caveman, our world has become more complex, and we're constantly running from far more than just a saber-toothed tiger. With pressures from our bosses; the Internet, which created a world in which everything is experienced in real time; and devices that have us on call 24/7, we've become addicted to producing more in less time. Instead of running from the tiger, we're running to beat the clock. As we sprint through life at breakneck speed, the originally protective stress response is activated far too often for non–life-threatening reasons. Over an extended period, the frequent activation of the stress response is harmful to our health.

With all the pressure we constantly confront, we're already on edge, and this gives us very little in reserve with which to respond to an unexpected life stress. Research shows that people with high emotional vitality who live life with fervor and purpose have developed ways to cope with life's sudden stressors. It's been speculated that their coping ability is why people with high emotional vitality are less likely to develop heart disease. We all need to find ways to cope with sudden life stress.

Acute, Sudden Stress

Stress comes in two main varieties: chronic and acute. Chronic stress is ongoing daily stress, like that experienced at work or in a difficult relationship. Acute stress is sudden and temporary, like that experienced in an earthquake or a tsunami. This chapter focuses on how to deal with acute stress and how to use B-R-E-A-T-H-E to break the stress cycle before it negatively affects your body.

The examples below illustrate how to recognize the body's response to stress and how to ultimately break the cycle by using your higher-functioning, rational brain rather than your primitive, impulsive, and emotional brain.

Stress: The Chain Reaction

Once you are exposed to the trigger of stress, a cascade of neuronal activity starts. Neurons are impulse-conducting cells that make up the brain, the spinal column, and the nerves. The first stop along the cascade is the primitive areas of the brain; then the more complex parts of the brain follow. This rush of activity also starts a set of brain-stem and midbrain responses that lead to a release of hormones, which causes an almost reflexive response.

Hormones released from the brain flood the bloodstream and stimulate the adrenal glands (a collection of specialized tissue that sits atop our kidneys), which release the stress hormones cortisol and adrenaline. This leads to classic signs and symptoms of stress, including dry mouth, dilated pupils, rapid heartbeat, fast and shallow breathing, and sweating.

In many instances, the initial chain reaction caused by stress is governed by the primitive emotional brain, so the reaction begins before we are even able to interpret it and figure out what's happening, which means that the higher brain suffers delayed notification. The higher brain is eventually notified of the hormonal storm, however, and then we can analyze and interpret the situation.

Once we acknowledge the stressful situation and are aware of our bodily changes and our physical response to stress, we can choose whether to respond with the higher brain, in a calm and productive fashion, or with the emotional brain, with impulsive and irrational behavior.

Let's say you're driving to work, and as you gradually merge onto the highway, someone cuts you off, blocking you from getting on the expressway. The rudeness and blatant disregard for driving etiquette infuriate you. At this point, you have an option: you can react reflexively and impulsively with your emotional brain and hunt the person down in a high-speed chase and risk going to jail; *or* your can listen to your body, feel your heart race and your rate of breathing increase, listen to the conversation between your heart and your brain, choose to dismiss the event as trivial, continue driving at a leisurely pace, and arrive at your destination mentally and physically intact.

That sounds pretty easy, but how does it work?

Even in the most maddening, frustrating, and difficult circumstances, you can choose not to become the victim and spiral out of control; instead, you can choose to say, "Duly noted—time to move on." You can learn to "flip a switch" in order to move from the emotional brain to the higher-functioning, reasoning brain. Flipping the switch involves two steps.

First, you hear the heart-brain conversation, which involves being aware of and recognizing the bodily response that has been caused by the stress hormones, which can include sweat on the brow, facial flushing, palpitations, or a dry mouth. The second step requires you to consciously choose to respond to the difficult situation in a productive, calm, and rational manner. Sometimes it is helpful to recall a pleasurable memory and to focus on your breathing.

Inside the brain, when you "flip the switch" from fight, flight, or freeze to *listen* (the conversation), *focus* (the retrieval of a pleasurable memory), and *breathe* (slowly), highly specialized nerve tissue known as *spindle neurons* are at work redirecting the train from the emotional track to the reasoning track.

Traumatic Events and Fears

Sometimes stress is created when we associate an uncomfortable situation with a traumatic and unpleasant memory. The caveman's negative memory was the saber-toothed tiger; yours might be an angry father. Consequently, an angry boss with a short fuse who's quick to raise his voice triggers unpleasant memories and consistently stresses you out.

Some traumatic events are so powerful that they leave a permanent mark on the nervous system, so that even the nerves carry a memory of the event. The sights, sounds, smells, and textures that were experienced during the stressful event are often seared into the memory bank and act as potent triggers for sudden stress.

The Trigger

Over time we develop irrational fears of things that are not life-threatening but that cause the same potentially harmful reflex: the flooding of stress hormones that would be released if we were running from someone who was pointing a gun at us.

The irrational fear is usually based on an uncomfortable and frequently old negative memory. Sometimes such memories are so emotionally charged and scarring that we deliberately try to forget the experiences. When we are exposed to a sight, a smell, a sound, or even a texture that is reminiscent of a traumatic event, the stress response can be activated, and the negative memory is retrieved at an unconscious level. Sometimes these memories rear their ugly heads and manifest themselves in the form of panic attacks, phobias, or irrational impulsive behaviors. Becoming involved in a road-rage incident or developing a panic attack while giving a public speech are examples of a stressful situation gone awry.

Other examples are a five-year-old boy who falls from a tree and develops a fear of heights, a seven-year-old girl who is afraid of dogs after being bitten by one, and a war veteran who flees for his life after hearing a motorcycle backfire, thinking it's a mortar shell. As we age, these patterns of behavior become more and more rigid. If these feelings and patterns remain unrecognized, the triggers become more and more emotionally charged.

Avoiding the Inevitable

A simple and common way to decrease the chance of experiencing one's triggers and uncomfortable feelings is to avoid them at all cost. The problem is that life doesn't always make it that easy. No matter how hard we try to avoid a triggering and uncomfortable situation, life throws us a curve ball. Despite all your effort to avoid elevators, you find yourself stuck on one between floors. All of a sudden, a man with a fear of heights spirals emotionally out of control when he's stuck in traffic on the Golden Gate Bridge, suspended thousands of feet above the ocean. The stress response is triggered, the stress hormones are released, the blood pressure soars, and the heart races.

In with the Good Memories and Out with the Bad

Modern neuroscience suggests that no matter how rigid and ingrained our behaviors and our fears are, we have the ability to change irrational and maladaptive behaviors that have been caused by stress. In a process known as *distraction*, or *reappraisal*, we can choose to think of or remember something that distracts us from the triggering situation.

This is one of the major benefits of the B-R-E-A-T-H-E technique. Instead of spiraling emotionally out of control, the fellow stuck in traffic on the Golden Gate Bridge thinks of how the water below reminds him of the deep blue beautiful flowing river that he imagines during his daily B-R-E-A-T-H-E exercise. Good memories and calming images are developed by regularly practicing the B-R-E-A-T-H-E technique. They are stored in our memory bank and are quickly retrievable and extremely useful for defusing a highly stressful and triggering situation.

Higher Brain: Lower Stress

When we react to stress with the primitive brain, we feel victimized, and the "Why me?" syndrome takes over. Yet even in the most stressful situations, we all have the ability to avoid self-destructing or spiraling emotionally out of control. When you practice the B-R-E-A-T-H-E technique, you will respond to stress more effectively. The unpredictable and uncontrollable nature of stress affects all of us, and no one is spared.

The way you respond to stress is entirely up to you. You can respond to stress in an impulsive and emotional way, or you can make a conscious effort to respond in a rational, calm, and productive way. The latter requires practice and skill, which is where B-R-E-A-T-H-E fits in. Recognizing and becoming aware of your body's response is the first step, and responding to the situation calmly and productively is the second step. This process requires using the higher brain rather than the primitive brain, and this becomes infinitely easier when you B-R-E-A-T-H-E.

From Fight, Flight, or Freeze to Listen, Focus, and Breathe

Recent research has led to the discovery of highly specialized cells known as *spindle neurons*, which are the air traffic controllers for the emotions in the brain. The cells are found in highest concentration in the part of the brain called the anterior cingulate cortex (ACC), which is activated during intense emotion.

The ACC functions as a filter or a lens and helps us to make sense of stressful situations. Acting as a gatekeeper, the ACC controls signals from the emotional brain (the amygdala) to the rational brain (the prefrontal cortex), using the special spindle neurons. The connection between the primitive and the higher parts of the brain is what allows us to have self-control in a stressful situation and to flip the switch and react calmly and coolly rather than impulsively and irrationally.

Here are two examples of how we can choose to respond to stress: one with the emotional primitive brain and one with the higher rational brain. Here is an emotional-brain scenario:

Emotional Primitive Brain Response

- Trigger: snakes
- Stressful emotion: fear
- Activation of amygdala, or primitive brain
- Retrieval of noxious memory: snake bite
- Activation of midbrain, or hypothalamus
- Release of stress hormones: adrenaline and cortisol
- Racing heart and soaring blood pressure
- Bodily symptoms: palpitations, sweating, feeling of impending doom
- Full-blown panic

You are literally scared stiff, so you freeze. This allows the snake to bite you, which further strengthens your fear of snakes.

Rational Brain Response

- Trigger: snakes
- Stressful emotion: fear

- Activation of amygdyla, or primitive brain
- Retrieval of noxious memory: snake bite
- Activation of midbrain, or hypothalamus
- Release of stress hormones: adrenaline and cortisol
- Racing heart and soaring blood pressure
- Activation of frontal cortex (rational brain)
- Acknowledgement of symptoms: hearing the conversation
- Activation of memory bank (hippocampus) and retrieval of pleasurable memory (distraction)
- Calm, focused, and productive behavior in response to the trigger

You see the snake and feel your heart racing. You realize that the snake, like you, is merely enjoying the warm sun. You acknowledge that it's not threatening; you continue walking, slowly and deliberately, away from the snake; and you avoid any problems by acting in a rational, productive, and reasonable manner.

Using B-R-E-A-T-H-E for Fast Help

The following examples illustrate how a triggering and emotionally charged situation can evoke an old negative memory and instantly stimulate the stress response. If we have developed the evolved part of our brain by using the B-R-E-A-T-H-E technique, we can rapidly retrieve positive memories for fast help in a stressful situation.

Even when we've been triggered and have become overwhelmed by our most feared stressors in life, we can quickly find a sense of calm using these helpful heart-healing images. We can't completely avoid stress in our lives, but we can definitely control how we respond to it.

When we react to stress and let our emotional primitive brain take over, we can quickly unravel and deal poorly with the situation. Yet if we choose to use our higher rational brain, we can deal with stress calmly and effectively, without ever breaking into a sweat. The trick is to make the switch from responding with the emotional brain to responding with the rational brain, and the B-R-E-A-T-H-E technique is what will enable you to make this switch.

Going Up, Not Down

Steve Carver was the senior hedge-fund manager at a large brokerage house in New York City. He purposely worked on the first floor of the large skyscraper because he secretly feared elevators. He dreaded the third Thursday of every month, because he sat on the board of directors and had to attend a meeting on the eighty-second floor, where he was required to present the current month's operating numbers to the rest of the board.

His fear was so great that he planned well in advance and would walk up *all eighty-two flights* to avoid a panic attack caused by a ride on the elevator. His irrational fear of elevators stemmed from a traumatic experience that had occurred when he was only four years old. While shopping with his mother, he got lost and meandered aimlessly onto the department-store elevator, where he and four others became trapped for several hours, until a team of firefighters rescued them.

This left an indelible mark on his psyche. Then, as a teenager, he once had a panic attack in an elevator and passed out. His head struck the ground, and he still had a scar above his right eyebrow as a painful reminder of the event.

One Thursday morning Steve was running late and was forced to take the elevator to the eighty-second floor. He was just beginning to panic when he noticed a beautiful painting hanging opposite the elevator doors inside the ornately decorated elevator. The painting was of a large sprawling oak tree. He became mesmerized by its beauty, and it reminded him of the oak tree on the river's edge that he imagined daily during his B-R-E-A-T-H-E routine. Steve's elevator phobia is a thing of the past.

Panicked: Sliver of Light

Roberta Potter, thirty-seven years old and in excellent physical shape, was a stay-at-home mom and part-time yoga instructor. Her days were exhausting. Some would say she had one of the most difficult jobs in the world: being the parent of two young children, an infant and a toddler, both in diapers.

Roberta performed superhuman feats on a daily basis, juggling shopping, running the house, cleaning, feeding two children, changing diapers, and making play dates. She did all of this on three to four hours of consistently interrupted sleep. She was exhausted and constantly sleep-deprived.

Roberta's only personal time was at seven-thirty in the evening, when her husband, a cardiologist, returned from work. With the kids finally asleep, she cherished this short, one hour of adult conversation. During this hour she often vented about the daily challenges of caring for two kids in diapers. The conversation also included her complaints about the enormous responsibility of caring for two children and the constant surveillance and monitoring that was required—all on little or no sleep.

Despite the daunting task of parenting two young children, the venting invariably ended with the acknowledgment by the two of them of the love they had for each other, which made it all seem worth it. Sipping a glass of wine and letting it all out to a pair of interested ears always seemed to make Roberta feel better. It empowered her to tackle the next day.

Roberta was an incredible mother with incredible mental fortitude, which she attributed to her yoga practice. Nevertheless, despite the focus that she had acquired from daily yoga, she was vulnerable to panic attacks. Though infrequent, these attacks were overwhelming, and she just couldn't seem to get a handle on them. They made it difficult for her to concentrate, which just made mothering all the more difficult.

Roberta knew the trigger for her panic attacks, however, so she avoided them like the plague. Small enclosed spaces, such as closets or rooms without windows, seemed to do the most triggering, so she made a conscious effort to avoid them altogether. (It's commonly believed that most cases of claustrophobia are generated from a childhood trauma in a closed-in space, such as a closet, or from having the feeling of being closed in.)

One day, while multitasking as usual with her infant in one arm and her toddler in the other, she attempted to start working on dinner. She was expecting relatives and friends and had planned a sit-down dinner. While preparing for the dinner party, she went to the walk-in pantry for a few ingredients, and as she entered the pantry, her three-year-old scurried in after her and pulled the door shut. As she heard the loud click of the child-safety lock they'd installed to protect the children, she realized that they were all locked in the pantry.

The pantry was dark, and the heavy door allowed little air in. A small crack of light entered through the top of the doorway. With her infant clutched in one arm and her toddler clinging to her leg, she frantically pushed on the door, to no avail. Her children, frightened by the dark, closed space, began to scream in unison.

Roberta was struck with panic as her worst fear became reality. Somehow she managed to call on her maternal instincts, and instead of spiraling out of control as she'd done so many times in the past, she felt everything slow down and she began to focus. Despite all the stress around her, with her children breathing shallowly and screaming and the air getting thicker by the moment, she sat on the ground with her back against the shelves and her legs pointed toward the door.

As she felt the typical beginning of a panic attack, she noticed the small sliver of light emanating through the top of the doorway. The light reminded her of the flickering radiance caused by the sun's reflection on the majestic river she envisioned during her daily B-R-E-A-T-H-E routine. Normally, she would already have begun to feel impending doom, as her panic attack developed, but instead she felt a peculiar and comforting sense of calm.

She pulled her infant close to her breast and held her toddler in her right arm, clutching them both tightly. Then she pulled her legs up close to her chest and imagined delivering a powerful outward thrust with her legs. After visualizing once, she coiled her legs into her chest tightly, took two deep breaths, and with a single mighty blow, kicked the heavy door open. A cool whisk of air swept through the pantry. She let out a massive sigh of relief and began weeping with joy. Her one- and three-year-old daughters began clapping for their mommy, their heroine.

Later Roberta thought of how experiences such as this had triggered panic attacks so many times in the past, and she marveled at her ability to stay focused and present despite being frightened. Instead of calling on old negative memories that led to spiraling out of control and into full-blown panic, she called on a positive thought and was able to weather and conquer the stressful storm. This experience allowed her to realize her ability to deal effectively with unexpected stress. With continued practice of the B-R-E-A-T-H-E technique, she was able to hone this skill, which ultimately allowed her to overcome her fear of small enclosed spaces.

Paddling Home: Breathing in Sync

Adriana Vargo had lived most of her life feeling left out; she had never felt part of any team or support group. She was a loner and attributed the difficulty she had making friends to her nearly crippling asthma. She wasn't able to play sports in school as other children did, and she was treated differently by her teachers.

Adriana's youth was plagued by visits to multiple doctors' offices and seasonal afflictions that seemed to be exacerbated by changes in the weather. In college she felt adventurous, and despite the fact that her symptoms worsened with exercise, she took a canoeing class and fell in love with both the water and the sport.

Once she moved to California after college, however, she never took up canoeing again. One morning, while Adriana was reading through the Sunday paper, she noticed an ad for canoeing lessons, and it sparked her pleasant college memories. The picture of the canoe inspired her to enroll at the local canoe club. As she became more adept and comfortable in her one-person canoe, she met a few avid rowers who convinced her to join a canoe team. Before Adriana knew it, she was rowing in canoeing competitions.

Her team was good and won many local races. Even though exercise typically made her asthma worse, Adriana noticed that when she was rowing on a team, she felt the power and synergy of the synchronized rhythm of her crew. She practiced B-R-E-A-T-H-E exercises each morning, and she noticed the same cadence and relaxing rhythm when rowing with her team.

One summer, while Adriana was on vacation in Hawaii, she decided to take a canoe out on the beautiful shores of Kauai. Once she was out on the water, she noticed that the air felt much denser than it did on shore. She noticed the thick humidity and mist on her arms and her shoulders. Suddenly she began wheezing and became short of breath. She knew that the sudden change in temperature was causing an asthma attack.

With each canoe stroke, Adriana felt slightly shorter of breath. She was out past the breakers and was concerned that she might not make it back to shore. For a moment it seemed as though she was beginning to black out, but as she looked down, she noticed the water as it caressed the sides of the canoe. She noticed a steady balmy Hawaiian breeze at her back and recalled the powerful flowing river from her B-R-E-A-T-H-E exercises. She began breathing in sync, as if she were with her team on the canoe, piercing through the water with great precision and force. The image of the river's strong current delivered her to shore safely. When she arrived, she was breathing comfortably.

Cooling Your Jets

It was a cool autumn day in Berlin when the majestic airbus took off from the Berlin-Brandenburg International Airport, headed for the Azores. Pierre Cousteau was a seasoned pilot and the captain of the flight, carrying three hundred tourists to their vacation destination.

Unknown to Pierre and his copilot, the aircraft had developed a leak in the fuel line to the right engine. During the course of the flight, the two men had noticed an imbalance between the fuel tanks in the left and the right wings of the aircraft, and they had attempted to remedy this by opening a valve between the tanks. This caused fuel to be wasted, though, because of the leak on the other side.

Pierre was able to glide the aircraft to a landing at Lajes Field (where there is a U.S. Air Force base) on Terceira Island in the Azores. The reported landing speed was much higher than normal. There were no fatalities, but there were minor injuries.

When Pierre lost power in the second engine, he panicked. He realized that without fuel, he'd lose all power to activate the landing gear. He felt his heart racing and beads of sweat forming on his forehead.

Suddenly, seemingly out of thin air, a strange voice with a Spanish accent came over his radio headset, informing him of a small military air base somewhere out in the middle of nowhere. In an instant he flipped the switch, and feelings of despair and angst turn to confidence and calm. Suddenly the impossible seemed possible. He took two large deep breaths and recalled a pleasurable childhood memory from when he was twelve years old, when he began learning to fly a crop duster over the vineyards in the south of France.

He recalled the feeling of gliding and making big exaggerated banking turns without power. The memory allowed him to focus and to execute an incredible landing that had never been done before. The entire flight crew and passengers safely deplaned, with only a few minor injuries.

When Pierre was interviewed after the miraculous event, he described being initially panicked but noted that a pleasurable memory involving his passion for flying allowed him to breathe, calm himself, concentrate, and focus. He explained that a ritual he practices—wherein he visualizes takeoff, flight, and landing before each trip—helped him to find a sense of calm in the harried situation. Even though the plane he was flying now was a hundred times bigger than the crop duster and was carrying three hundred people, he thought of how the planes he had flown were more similar than different.

Thus, a single pleasurable memory of his childhood instantaneously changed his outlook and helped him to flip the switch. His recollection of flying over the beautiful countryside of southern France reminded him of his passion for flying and was instrumental in helping him to focus and remain in the moment. He simply imagined that the jet without power was no different from the small planes on which he had learned to fly.

Full Count, Bases Loaded

Great athletes have an uncanny ability to perform their best when they are under enormous pressure.

Instead of folding when they are asked for the game-winning hit, the near-perfect dive, or a score of ten to clinch the medal, professional athletes are able to flip the switch, focus, and execute.

The ability to perform under pressure when the stakes are high enables many professional athletes to make the successful transition into business, consulting, coaching, lecturing, or teaching. They seem to be blessed with something special that they're able to call on when they're challenged. Even more impressive is their ability to replicate the skill time and again under pressure. They seem to possess a special skill that's foreign to the rest of us.

Yet as humans we are all born with the same "software"; believe it or not, all of us have the same potential ability as an athlete. The key is to understand the wiring of the system and how to flip the switch. Even when we are overwhelmed, we all have the capacity to find calm in the eye of the most wicked and powerful storms.

Manny Nagel, a baseball player, shows how he has successfully flipped the switch. Instead of considering the enormous pressure and the tremendous responsibility on his shoulders—his teammates, their families who had traveled long distances to be at the game, his devoted coach, his fans, and his career—he triumphs in this stressful situation.

When called to perform, he resorts to his higher brain rather than his primitive one. With a full count and bases loaded, he steps out of the batter's box, signals the umpire to regroup, and collects his thoughts. He scans the stadium and feels the vibration and roar of the raucous crowd, which begins to chant his name in unison and clap. The sound is almost deafening.

Manny's career and the future success or failure of his team will be determined by this one final pitch.

As he steps back into the batter's box, he recalls a tip his swing coach gave him last week in batting practice to level his arms and increase his swing speed. He imagines the bat hitting the ball and then takes two big deep breaths, extending his exhalation. Next, he tucks the extra material of his shirt under his armpit, just as his coach recommended. His heart rate slows, and he feels as though he can see the ball in the pitcher's glove before the pitcher releases it. He sees the ball leaving the hand of the pitcher. He sees it in exquisite detail, and despite the fact that it is traveling at a speed of ninety miles per hour, he watches as his bat strikes the ball perfectly, sending it high over the center field wall.

B-R-E-A-T-H-E
Fast Help When You're Overwhelmed

All these stories are examples of how the B-R-E-A-T-H-E technique can help to defuse an overwhelmingly stressful situation and change an outcome almost instantaneously.

We all have the ability to deal effectively with life-threatening or seemingly life-threatening situations. If Pierre, for example, had let his emotions take over by thinking of the most common outcomes in the dismal history of unsuccessful landings, his outcome would have been disastrous.

Instead, in a split second he tapped into a pleasurable memory that helped him to focus and catch his breath. This memory allowed him to concentrate and draw on his extraordinary flying skills, which helped him to execute a literally death-defying feat and ultimately bring the jet and its three hundred passengers to safety. He was able to make a switch from the emotional brain to the rational brain because he had practiced thousands of times before.

When Pierre first felt stressed, he noticed the physiological changes in his body. The sweat on his brow and his racing heart were his cues to participate in the heart-brain conversation. Two deep breaths and extended exhalations later, he recalled a pleasurable memory, which helped him to focus and safely land the jet.

Inside his brain, something fascinating was taking place. The spindle neurons, which he developed using the B-R-E-A-T-H-E technique, helped him to bridge the neural activity from the primitive brain to the higher brain, which helped him to act calmly, rationally, and effectively in a truly life-threatening situation.

A simple pleasurable and positive memory retrieved in the moment of need served to instantaneously "flip the switch" in him from despair to hope.

Similarly, Roberta, locked in the pantry with her two children, used the light at the top of the doorway to recall the sun's reflection on the river, the image she had been using in her B-R-E-A-T-H-E practice. Steve, with his elevator phobia, recalled an oak tree, and Adriana, on the brink of an asthma attack in a canoe, recalled the powerful current of the river.

These memories, all consciously chosen and recalled, were formed by practicing the B-R-E-A-T-H-E technique and were readily available in a pinch.

Just as a panic attack is triggered, for example, when someone associates the odor of gasoline with an explosion in childhood and the resulting burns, a positive, relaxing, and calming memory will have an equal and opposite effect on our physiology.

The B-R-E-A-T-H-E technique will allow you to develop this ability and to focus and execute when you're stressed—and maybe even when you're in a life-threatening situation.

9

Is Heart Disease Contagious?

Sara Warren suddenly felt sweaty and light-headed as the doctor explained her father's critical condition to her. Later, she remembered the words "he had a serious heart attack" being spoken by the cardiologist. She vaguely recalled her stomach starting to churn and the near-blinding bright lights of the ICU going dim. She remembered everything looking black and white, and in the same instant, the loud, obnoxious bells and alarms in the hectic ICU became muffled and distorted. The next thing she saw was the hard shiny hospital floor, which broke her fall.

She woke with her family huddled around her bed and anxiously peering down at her. Even more puzzling to her were the bandages covering her chest. "Where am I, and what are those?" she asked.

On receiving the news of her father's nearly fatal heart attack from the cardiologist, Sara had become overwhelmed and passed out. Unbeknown to Sara, her heart had stopped, and a Code Blue team was called. She was quickly resuscitated. Her ECG revealed a rare type of arrhythmia that, when triggered by an emotional event, can cause a lethal arrhythmia. The ECG also revealed a rare form of ventricular tachycardia known as Brugada syndrome, which was triggered by the unexpected and shocking news of her father's condition.

Two People, One Heart

You don't catch heart disease like the common cold. You can't get it by visiting someone in the cardiac ICU or by close contact with someone who has heart disease. Yet the worry and anxiety experienced by friends and family after a loved one suffers a heart attack or an acute cardiac event can be intense. In fact, the high anxiety internalized by family members for the affected individual is at times so powerful and emotionally charged that they themselves became at risk for developing cardiac symptoms—giving real meaning to the terms *worried sick* and *heartbroken.*

As a cardiologist I frequently witness how the emotional bonds for loved ones are so strong and so deep that our concerns and worries about family members and friends become harmful to our own hearts. It's almost as if heart disease or cardiac events were contagious.

The pain experienced by a mother or a father before, during, and after a child's heart attack sweeps like a wave through the family. In a blink of an eye, the entire family and its support group frequently experience chest pain, difficulty breathing, or palpitations. I call this phenomenon *one heart.* People, especially a family, are connected in such a way that the cardiovascular health and well-being of one is related to the cardiovascular health and well-being of another.

When a family member gets sick due to the emotional stress that has been caused by the acute illness of a loved one, it's called the *caregiver effect*. The most severe form of this contagious-like phenomenon is known as the *widower effect* and occurs when a spouse is hospitalized. When that occurs, the partner's risk of death increases significantly and remains elevated for up to two years. The greatest risk for the partner occurs within thirty days of the hospitalization or death of the spouse.

Researchers examined heart-risk factors in family members of cardiac patients and found that those who provided all or most of a patient's care had higher levels of risk factors for heart disease than noncaregivers did. Those who reported higher caregiver strain after six months were more likely to be depressed than those who provided less or no care.

There is growing evidence that stress and depression play an important role in the development of cardiovascular disease:

- Caregivers exhibit exaggerated cardiovascular responses to stressful conditions, which puts them at greater risk than noncaregivers for the development of cardiovascular syndromes such as high blood pressure or heart disease.
- Women who provide care to an ill or disabled spouse are more likely to report a personal history of high blood pressure, diabetes, and high levels of cholesterol.
- Women who spend nine or more hours a week caring for an ill or a disabled spouse increase their risk of heart disease twofold.

Additional studies found that educating caregivers and family members of hospitalized cardiac patients about their own heart risks and providing them information about a heart-healthy diet improved their eating habits after six weeks.

It's important to recognize that the stress that is felt when a loved one falls ill is the same as the stress you experience when you are pressured for time, stuck in traffic, speaking in public, or strapped for cash. Your body doesn't know the difference, so it responds in the same potentially destructive way. The same hormones are released, causing damage to our delicate cardiac tissue.

When you are worrying about a spouse or a loved one who is undergoing a major operation, who has just had a heart attack, or who has recently been diagnosed with an illness, it's more important than ever to listen to the conversation between your heart and your brain, pay attention to your body's response to this powerful stressor, and B-R-E-A-T-H-E.

Staying focused and calm and using the B-R-E-A-T-H-E technique will help you to cope with this extremely challenging situation so that you can provide the necessary support and compassion for your loved one while also protecting your own health and well-being.

A Slippery Slope

When a loved one is diagnosed with a sudden cardiac event, a slippery slope arises. After a heart attack, people are at higher risk of developing depression, which is associated with poorer outcomes and higher mortality. Patients who are at highest risk for depression are those with "lonely hearts" or no social support. The converse is true as well. Patients with more social support—loved ones and friends who are available to them after a heart attack—are at much lower risk for depression and have lower cardiac mortality.

Yet although strong family support is essential for preventing depression and lonely heart syndrome in the post–heart attack patient, too much concern and worry by the family can lead to the caregiver effect.

Studies show that the presence of a supportive person during stress is beneficial to health by lessening one's cardiovascular response to a stressor. Better social support after a heart attack has led to better recovery and improved mortality for those patients, compared to patients with little or no social support. Being isolated or alone after a heart attack increases your risk of depression, which has been directly linked to increased cardiac mortality.

The following stories illustrate the powerful emotional bonds of family, the potentially harmful one-heart phenomenon, and the cardio-protective effect of the B-R-E-A-T-H-E technique for family members.

Slam-dunked

The world will never know a prouder single mother than Sandra Hamilton. As she watched her son Larry (a high school All-American basketball player) play in his final championship game, she watched him make a fast break, beat the defense to the hoop, and, as if suspended in the air, execute an amazing dunk, which won the game and brought the packed house of fans to their feet with a deafening ovation.

While the crowd continued a maddening ovation for the highly recruited high school phenomenon, he suddenly fell to the cold gymnasium floor. His mother reflexively sprinted from her front-row seat to aid her son. The sudden stress precipitated a heart attack in Sandra at the same time that her son Larry lay lifeless on the floor. Mother and son were both resuscitated on the scene and rushed to the nearby hospital.

Larry was diagnosed with hypertrophic obstructive cardio-myopathy (HOCM), a thickening of the walls of the heart and the same disease that killed legendary basketball greats Hank Gathers and Reggie Lewis as well as dozens of other great athletes. Four of the main arteries to Sandra's heart were almost totally blocked from a lifetime of unhealthy diet and bad lifestyle choices. Mother and son were both brought into surgery, where Larry received an ICD—a small implantable cardioverter-defibrillator that jump-starts the heart with a jolt of electricity when an arrhythmia is detected—and Sandra had an emergency bypass. Both had successful procedures and were discharged a few days later.

In a very happy ending to a potentially tragic story, Larry went on to become the highly successful coach of a college basketball team and a frequent speaker on the subject of heart disease to young athletes. Sandra lost more than a hundred pounds, became physically active, and currently teaches yoga.

Shocked

Sam Jensen, an elderly man, was working in his garden trying to remove some old roots from a tree when he accidentally cut himself with his axe and began bleeding profusely. Too weak to move, he began calling for his wife, Dot, who was in the house and anxiously waiting for him to finish so that he could drive her to her cardiologist's appointment. Dressed and ready, with her arms folded and her foot nervously tapping the floor, she heard her husband's faint cry for help coming from the backyard.

Dot walked into the garden and saw Sam lying in a large pool of bright red blood. She clutched her chest and fell unconscious. Finally, her husband dragged himself to the workbench in the garage, where he'd put his cell phone, and called 911.

Later, at the hospital, as the final suture was being sewn to close Sam's laceration, he learned that his wife was in stable condition in the cardiac care unit, where the records of her ICD were evaluated and discovered to have delivered five lifesaving shocks to correct Dot's life-threatening arrhythmia. When these records were checked against the paramedics' notes, it was discovered that the stress Dot experienced from her husband's injury had triggered her life-threatening arrhythmia, which caused her ICD to appropriately shock her.

Help!

Marisa Aguna had been Marshall Johnston's housekeeper for thirty-five years. She'd originally been hired to help around the house after his wife's death, but she and her three children had actually become Marshall's surrogate family. Marshall was a vigorous eighty-year-old who acted as if he were going on fifty. He exercised regularly and insisted on being actively involved in his successful dry cleaning business.

During the thirty-five years that she'd worked for him, Marisa had moved from being his housekeeper to his bookkeeper, personal assistant, and occasional lover. The bond between them was so strong that Marisa, her children, and Marshall were like family.

One afternoon, after shopping for groceries, as she approached the house she noticed Marshall's car sitting in the garage as if it hadn't been moved from the night before, and she got a funny feeling that something wasn't quite right.

A rush of anxiety overwhelmed her, and horrible thoughts about the well-being of Marshall raced through her head. She frantically riffled through her purse for the keys to the palatial colonial home. She ran up the steps to the front porch, opened the door, and began yelling, "Marshall, Marshall, are you okay?" Her voice echoed throughout the large foyer and the rest of the house, but she received no answer. As she looked up the large spiral staircase, she saw Marshall lying on the floor at the top and mumbling, "Help, Marisa, help!"

She grabbed her cell phone and called 911. As she ran upstairs toward Marshall, she noticed that with each step she had more difficulty breathing. As she reached the top of the stairs she felt a sudden constricting squeezing in her chest. She clenched the banister to brace herself from falling, and as she looked down at a nearly lifeless Marshall Johnston, she collapsed beside him.

Here are some interesting statistics:

- Elderly spousal caregivers (ages 66–96) who experience caregiving-related stress have a 63 percent higher mortality rate than noncaregivers of the same age.
- In 2006, the hospitalization of an elderly spouse was found to be associated with an increased risk of caregiver death.

Minutes later, help arrived, and the four paramedics who raced up the staircase found two patients gasping for breath, lying next to each other. They were rushed to the hospital, where Marshall was evaluated and diagnosed with severe calcific aortic stenosis and Marisa was diagnosed with severe three-vessel coronary artery disease. Marshall underwent a surgery the next morning for aortic valve replacement, and Marisa received triple bypass surgery. Eventually, both recovered, and less than a year later they were married, with Marisa's three grown children in attendance.

Till Death Do Us Part: Lovers' Quarrel Taken to Heart

Suzie and Greg Lewis had been together for thirty years and married for twenty-seven. They'd put three children through college and were settling into a new and more relaxed retirement lifestyle. Suzie had worked for twenty-five years as a court reporter, and Greg had retired from thirty-five years of service with the San Francisco Police Department.

They loved each other deeply, but they just couldn't seem to move beyond a common pattern of arguing that defined all their years together. It seemed that every time they rode in the same car, a heated argument would ensue. Realizing that this was a sensitive trigger, they had avoided riding in the same car for years, so they often traveled to places in separate cars just to avoid conflict. Now, however, newly retired and anticipating frequent travel and common activities, they were forced to do the unthinkable and ride together.

One sunny summer day they started a short trip with the best of intentions. They even acknowledged before they left that riding together had always been an issue, so they would both do their best to refrain from the old dysfunctional pattern. After all, this was just going to be a three-hour drive to the Monterey Aquarium.

Predictably, it only took thirty minutes to trigger the old arguing pattern. Suddenly their dreams of rest and relaxation were shattered and replaced with anger and resentment.

The argument started as it always did, with Suzie commenting on how closely Greg was following the car in front of them. Greg, as usual, took this observation personally and began yelling,

"If you don't like the way I drive, then you drive." The argument quickly degenerated further and included expletives and name-calling. Greg's pattern was to scream, and Suzie's was to become silent and feel furious inside.

There are two important points to keep in mind:

1. Marital arguing style can negatively impact our hearts.
2. In a ten-year study, the women who kept quiet and didn't speak their minds were four times more likely to die during the time of the study than the women who always told their husbands how they felt.

As the fight grew more heated, Greg found it more and more difficult to concentrate on the road. He pulled over at the next rest area, and as he started getting out of the car, he felt sweaty and queasy, as if he were going to throw up. He pushed open the door, stood up, clutched his chest, and, with Suzie still sitting in the car stewing, he fell to his knees. She opened her door and got out, and as she ran around to his side of the car she felt light-headed, became short of breath, and had rapid palpitations that felt as though her heart was going to jump out of her chest.

When she reached her husband, she saw that his face had turned a bluish hue, so Suzie grabbed her cell phone and frantically called 911. Paramedics were on the scene within minutes, and once they'd stabilized her husband and loaded him into the waiting ambulance, she told one of them about her symptoms. The paramedic checked her pulse, which was racing at more than two hundred beats a minute, and a field ECG confirmed a tachycardia. A second ambulance was quickly summoned, and Suzie and Greg were both brought to a nearby emergency room.

Marital arguing patterns have been studied, and certain patterns of arguing have been proven to be cardio-toxic.

Greg is a classic example of how rage and hostility can precipitate a cardiac event. Hostility has been associated with acute cardiac events, particularly in men.

Suzie is another classic example of how an arguing pattern can contribute to a cardiac event. Studies now suggest that women who repress their feelings and harbor resentment toward their husbands instead of expressing their emotions (in a constructive manner, of course) are particularly prone to cardiac events.

These stories illustrate the powerful emotional bonds we share with family members or other loved ones. Profound concern, empathy, and compassion for a heart-disease patient can activate the stress response and cause harm to one's own heart. We need to be conscious and aware of the one-heart phenomenon.

On hundreds of occasions, I've experienced entire families flying in from all over the world after a family member's cardiac event, and I have witnessed how intense worry passes from member to member in a chain reaction. Although we should be careful of our own hearts in this situation, we also need to be sensitive to the needs of the affected loved one. Understanding the delicate balance between internalizing the pain and suffering of our loved ones and the potential harm of isolation and loneliness to the cardiac patient is crucial for getting us through this challenging life stress. Almost all of us will be faced with this reality, so it is important to be aware of it.

The B-R-E-A-T-H-E technique is appropriate for both parties. For the patient, it serves as an educational and healing exercise, and for family members it serves to educate and protect their vulnerable hearts.

B-R-E-A-T-H-E
The Family Tree Exercise

This B-R-E-A-T-HE exercise is designed to help those dealing with the stress created by the illness of a family member or other loved one. The focus of this exercise and the intention of the meditation is the family tree and how you can help the tree grow by rewarding yourself with this pleasurable exercise.

Begin

Begin your exercise in your warm, cozy, and familiar place. Wear loose-fitting clothing and settle comfortably in your favorite chair or sofa. Always start your exercise by listening to the conversation. Remember that your heart and your brain are connected and in constant communication. Listen to your heart.

Take a deep breath in through your nose and let it out through your mouth. Count s-l-o-w-l-y to seven. Notice that when you take in a deep breath, your heart rate slightly increases, and as you exhale, your heart rate decreases. Take a few more breaths and notice this trend: in, your heart rate increases; out, your heart rate decreases. The more you practice, the better you will get at hearing your heartbeat. This is excellent proof that you are participating in the conversation.

As you begin, focus on your heart and clear your mind of any other thoughts. Liken this exercise to working out different muscles in the gym. Instead of working your back, your shoulders, or your biceps, look at this exercise as exercising and developing your heart-brain connection.

Relax

Remember that the relaxation response is a state of deep relaxation that is the opposite of the fight-or-flight response. You can reach this state by deep breathing. It is comfortable, soothing, and nurturing for your heart. Breathing in and out causes changes in the heart rate. When you take a deep breath in, you are activating the sympathetic nervous system, which causes your heart rate to speed up. When you exhale, count to seven, like the number of letters in B-R-E-A-T-H-E. This extended exhalation activates the parasympathetic nervous system and slows the heart rate by sending signals from your brain to your heart on a highway called the vagus nerve. This fluctuation or variability of the heart rate is good for the heart.

Walk the path of relaxation and flow (see chapter 4). The sights and sounds are soothing, and as you take each step you become more conscious of your breathing. Your breathing and walking are in sync, and with each step you become more and more relaxed. You recognize this path and associate it with feelings of warmth, contentment, and peace, and you feel as though you've walked this path thousands of times before. The soft dust on your feet, the warm sun on your shoulders, and the fresh, clean, crisp air make you feel comfortable, secure, and relaxed. Each step is familiar, comforting, and soothing.

Envision

As you sit in a comfortable position at the foot of a majestic river, peer across and revel in the beauty of a massive oak in front of you. Think of how the tree and your family both started out very small, as just a tiny sapling. Over time the small bud grew, and with the constant flow of the river, the tree matured and grew into a large beautiful oak. Think of how the fertile soil is like the love of your family, which nurtured you throughout your life. The consistent and abundant flow of the river is like the consistent love and compassion that you have for each of your family members.

Appreciate all of the tree's parts, from its deep sprawling roots, which remind you of your family tree and genealogical origins, to its broad-based trunk, its strong winding branches, and its beautiful leaves. Imagine how each part is dependent yet separate and serves a different purpose. Each part, from the leaves and the trunk to the branches and the bark, requires its own basking in the sun and its own nourishment. Appreciate how all the parts, though connected, are also uniquely separate and individual. Imagine how the tree, just like your family, provides security and protection for the local wildlife (you). The leaves, for example, provide shade for the squirrels and the deer, and the branches provide shelter for the birds.

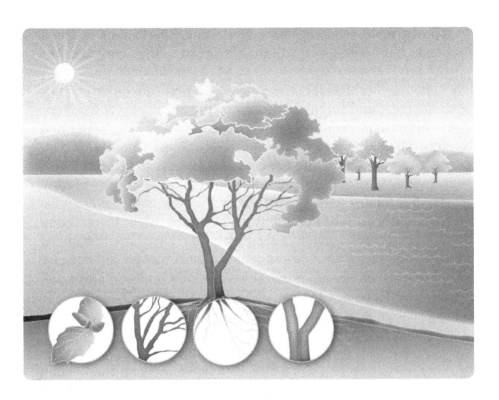

Apply

Make a mental connection and apply how the river resembles healthy arteries and a smoothly flowing electrical system. Imagine the tree to be your family tree, strong, connected, and secure. Note how the beautiful vegetation around you represents your healthy heart. Listen to the sounds around you. The gentle breeze blowing in the trees, the chirping of the birds, and the sound of the distant waterfall resemble your heart—constant, rhythmic, and powerful.

Treat

View this exercise as a special treatment for yourself. You are deserving of this pleasurable and therapeutic time. The exercise is pleasurable, relaxing, and rejuvenating. This is not a chore or a task. Before long you will look forward to this work and feel like a runner who experiences a high from running.

Remember that this exercise, when performed correctly, is therapeutic and serves to decrease your heart rate, lower your blood pressure, and lower your vascular tone. The deeper and more relaxed you become, the more protective and effective is the therapy. Meditation and exercises such as B-R-E-A-T-H-E technique are therapeutic: they lower the levels of cardio-toxic hormones such as cortisol and adrenaline. This exercise increases heart-rate variability and low fluctuations in heart rate (low heart-rate variability) in patients who have been diagnosed with poor cardiovascular outcomes. Recall that guided imagery bolsters the immune system, lowers blood pressure and heart rate, and decreases anxiety.

Heal

When using the B-R-E-A-T-H-E technique, imagine the healing properties of relaxation. Your deep breathing helps you to train the nerves that connect the brain and the heart and has a calming and slowing effect on your heart rate. This exercise will reduce stress and make you feel better, which will enhance healing in your body. It will allow you to downshift so that your engine can cool and idle for a while. Imagine that the warm sun on your shoulders causes your blood vessels to dilate, further improving flow and thus healing your electrical system. Store the heart-healing metaphors in your memory so they can be quickly retrieved to help protect and heal your heart in a stressful situation.

End

As you end your B-R-E-A-T-H-E exercise, recall all of the heart-healing metaphors and summarize their significance and their relationship to your healing heart. As you end your exercise, think of the intention and topic of this focused relaxation exercise. It's you and your family, the tree, and its many healthy branches. Think about how this special exercise time helped you to relax and rejuvenate so that you can care for them better when you are needed. As you end your exercise, you will become aware of your surroundings and feel energized. Your heart is strong, rhythmic, and unobstructed like the river. You and your family will be fine.

10

Stress and Cardiac Zebras

Many centuries ago, Friar William of Occam declared that common things are common, uncommon things are uncommon, and the simple and obvious answer is generally the right one. Over the years his reasoning has come to be known as Occam's razor and is frequently expressed by the statement that when you hear the sound of beating hooves, it's probably horses—not zebras.

Every day I'm called to the emergency room to see patients who have come in with chest pain, and almost always the beating hooves turn out to be blocked arteries. On rare occasions, however, I'll find evidence of an unusual murmur or a peculiar finding on an echocardiogram or an X-ray that indicates I've encountered a zebra instead of a horse.

Cardiac Zebras

In this chapter you'll learn that stress has an even more powerful negative impact on less common, but equally stress-sensitive, cardiac conditions. As in previous chapters, you'll notice a common theme: the toxic stress hormones exacerbate a specific ailing heart part for each uncommon and zebralike cardiac condition.

The stories below will describe how stress adversely affects the four heart parts, though in far less common cardiac disorders:

- The heart muscle in Chagas disease
- The arterial system in Marfan syndrome
- The electrical system in arrhythmogenic right ventricular dysplasia (ARVD)
- The heart valves in rheumatic mitral stenosis

Kiss and Tell: Stress and Chagas Disease

Palo Carlos was a Brazilian soccer enthusiast who dreamed of someday being as famous as his hero Pelé. Although he never got a chance to see Pelé play, Palo felt a special kinship with the famed soccer star. Common to both was their birthplace, a small village on the outskirts of Rio de Janeiro, and an obsession with futbol, or, as it is known in the United States, soccer.

Palo's dedication and commitment to the game included his daily ritual of dribbling his soccer ball to and from school. He weaved in and out of traffic and over the partially paved and tortuous dirt streets as if his ball were just another appendage. This inseparable connection, his constant study of the game, and his dedication to practice led to extraordinary footwork and exceptional soccer skills.

Finally, one day his phenomenal soccer skills were recognized by a talent scout, and he was recruited to play for a professional soccer team in the United States.

After flying to the United States and while riding the bus to the new apartment provided by the U.S. United Soccer Team, Palo noticed that he was having difficulty swallowing. In the next few days he felt short of breath several times while he was lying flat, but he attributed both symptoms to feeling nervous and excited about his dream coming true, his new career as a professional soccer player.

Attempting to impress his coaches, he pulled an all-nighter the night before the first full practice and memorized the entire hundred-page playbook. The next morning, sleep-deprived, dehydrated, and toxically caffeinated, he stepped onto the soccer field for the first time and was startled by the loud, demanding voice of his coach, which seemed to echo through the stadium. He suddenly felt his heart flutter, then he clutched his chest and collapsed on the perfectly manicured field. A trainer quickly initiated CPR, and a nearby defibrillator was placed on his chest. Palo was diagnosed with ventricular tachycardia, a lethal heart rhythm.

The coach, whose loud baritone voice had startled Palo and triggered the event, quickly called 911 on his cell phone, and following the instructions for the defibrillator, quickly began administering shocks. Each shock lifted Palo's two-hundred-pound body off the turf like a rag doll. Finally, after the third attempt, a regular rhythm was restored.

It took seven minutes for the rescue workers to arrive, and Palo's oxygen-deprived brain cells were already beginning to die. The paramedics continued CPR, trying to correct the deadly rhythm that had started in his left ventricle. Palo was lucky, for unlike six hundred thousand Americans who die suddenly each year because of a cardiac event, his life was saved by an astute and quick-acting coach.

Palo was brought to a nearby hospital. In the emergency room, blood tests and chest radiographs confirmed the diagnosis of congestive heart failure, and electrocardiograms revealed multiple recordings of a potentially lethal heart rhythm known as ventricular tachycardia.

The physician ordered an echocardiogram and a cardiology consultation. The echocardiogram revealed an abnormally enlarged and misshapen left ventricle.

Cardiologist's Analysis: A Bug Bite That Kills

When the cardiologist arrived, Palo was resting comfortably on an ICU gurney. An IV infused the powerful drug amiodarone into his left arm; this quieted his irritable heart and suppressed the lethal cardiac rhythm.

The cardiologist obtained a thorough history, which included questions about childhood illnesses and prior hospitalizations. When she asked about recent symptoms, Palo described his trouble swallowing, his shortness of breath, and his intermittent palpitations.

The astute cardiologist asked Palo about any insect bites or exposure to what are called kissing bugs. He recalled when an elementary teacher had lectured the students about an outbreak of kissing bugs, and he remembered that this outbreak had affected his entire family and most of his classmates. He told the cardiologist that he had been bitten in the face, and he remembered his eyes becoming extremely itchy and swollen.

This history was the piece of the puzzle that allowed the cardiologist to clinch the diagnosis. Using Occam's razor, she realized that all of Palo's symptoms kept leading her to one diagnosis: Chagas disease, which is caused by a parasite transmitted by the bite of the kissing bug. A special blood test confirmed the presence of the parasite in Palo and sealed the diagnosis of Chagas disease. Palo's echocardiogram's findings were also consistent with Chagas disease: dilation of both upper chambers of the heart (biatrial enlargement); scarring and thickening of the tip, or apex, of the heart; and leaky heart valves.

The Cause of Chagas Disease

Chagas disease is a tropical disease caused by the parasite *Trypanosoma cruzi*, which is transmitted to humans by the bite of the Reduviid bug, or kissing bug. The symptoms of Chagas disease vary over the course of the infection and in the years that follow. As the disease progresses, serious chronic symptoms can appear, including cardiac and intestinal problems.

Chagas disease occurs exclusively in the Americas, particularly in the poor rural areas of Mexico and of Central and South America. It is estimated that 8 to 11 million people in Mexico, Central America, and South America have Chagas disease, and most of them are unaware of their infection. It's even been postulated that Charles Darwin suffered and died from complications related to Chagas disease.

At night the Reduviid bugs, which harbor the parasite, hide in the thatched rooftops and bite people's faces while they are sleeping—hence the name kissing bugs. The infected person automatically scratches the affected site, which often spreads the parasite into the eyes. The most recognized early symptom of Chagas disease is Romana's sign (or chagoma), a swelling of the eyelids near the bite wound.

Repeated studies demonstrate that years or even decades after the infection, 30 percent of infected people will have developed medical problems that involve the nervous, cardiac, and digestive symptoms. Two-thirds of the 30 percent will develop cardiac damage that leads to congestive heart failure, heart rhythm abnormalities, and even sudden death. The other one-third of the 30 percent will develop digestive diseases such as a severely dilated colon or a dilated esophagus accompanied by severe weight loss.

If untreated, Chagas disease can be fatal, in most cases due to heart muscle damage. Chagas disease also damages the electrical system of the heart, causing both slow rhythms and various degrees of heart blockage as well as fast heart rhythms, such as ventricular tachycardia and ventricular fibrillation.

Stressors

The triggers of Palo's cardiac event included a startle response to the coach's loud and sudden voice, dehydration, sleep deprivation, physical exertion, and caffeine. All these stressors triggered the release of stress hormones, which increased the rate and irritability of Palo's heart. In the setting of Chagas disease, this caused a nearly fatal episode of ventricular tachycardia.

Our Patient

Prior to being discharged from the hospital, Palo was treated with a fancy device known as a combination pacemaker-ICD, and he was prescribed medications that made his heart beat slower and maintain a regular rhythm.

Palo used two B-R-E-A-T-H-E techniques, the Fallen Tree Exercise and the Cherry Blossom Exercise, regularly, and this helped him to recover. The visual metaphors in these exercises helped him to envision a strong healthy heart with unobstructed flow. In addition, his doctor recommended physical exams and echocardiograms for his entire family due to the prevalence of the disease in endemic countries in Latin and South America and all of sub-Saharan Africa.

Palo recovered successfully from his treatment. He stopped playing competitive soccer, as instructed by his doctors, but he is using his experience and his expertise to forge a successful coaching career. He often attributes his coaching success to the B-R-E-A-T-H-E technique, which he routinely teaches to all his players. His motto is "Envision, concentrate, focus, and execute on the field."

Death and Taxes: Marfan Syndrome

Natalie Ingall was a world-class sprinter and an Olympic gold medalist. After her final lap around the track, she landed a position with a high-profile sports psychology company, which specialized in mentally preparing professional athletes for competition.

Natalie had an exceptionally prosperous and busy year in 2005. TV commercials, sports commentating, and even a minor part in a movie kept her moving at a clip almost as fast as when she was competing.

All these exciting opportunities caused enormous pressure on her schedule; beating the clock took on a whole new meaning for Natalie. Juggling her travel, consulting, sports commentating, and public appearances exhausted her much of the time. The biggest difference between her new life and when she'd been competing was that back then she'd at least always been able to reward herself with short breaks, such as spas, massages, reading, and relaxation. Her new frenzied lifestyle was quite different; it seemed to have only one gear and no option to downshift.

On a cross-country trip, she developed a cough and a fever, which lingered for a month. She finally visited her regular doctor, who ordered a chest X-ray that confirmed her suspicion: Natalie had pneumonia.

In addition, the doctor had noticed something unusual and unexpected: Natalie had a dilated aorta. The aorta is a large garden hose–sized artery that carries blood from the main pumping chamber (the left ventricle) to the brain and the rest of the body.

The aorta is divided into three main parts:

1. The ascending aorta, which exits from the main pump and carries blood in an upward direction toward the brain

2. The transverse aorta, which crosses from the front of the heart to the back and is curved like the top of a candy cane

3. The descending aorta, which carries blood downward to the rest of the body and looks like the bottom of a candy cane

On Natalie's chest X-ray, her ascending aorta appeared wider than usual. The doctor pointed this out to Natalie and explained that an abnormal dilation of this part of the aorta may represent an aneurysm and that further testing to confirm this diagnosis was needed immediately. The doctor ordered a CT scan of Natalie's chest to further define the extent of the aneurysm and instructed Natalie to walk immediately down the hall to the radiology suite. She also asked Natalie two more things: how tall she was and to please hold her hands out sideways as far as she could reach. After carefully examining Natalie's fingers, the doctor jotted information down in her notes.

Natalie was shocked and confused about the bad news, yet all she could think of in this desperate moment was being late for her appointment with her agent. She apologized to the doctor, saying that she was thankful for her thoroughness and genuine concern but that she would be unable to get the test done right away because of a previous engagement. Half honoring the doctor's recommendation, she agreed to schedule the test the next day.

On the way down the staircase, she considered the magnitude and the implications of the things her doctor had just told her. She kept thinking to herself, "Aortic aneurysm—no way, I'm an Olympic athlete! How can this be possible?"

Late for her meeting, she ran out the door and hailed a taxi. During the frantic ride through the bustling city, with multiple traffic lights, honking horns, and bottleneck traffic, she got an unexpected phone call from her accountant. His tone was apologetic, and much to her surprise he proceeded to explain that she owed far more money on her taxes than she expected.

This caused Natalie to panic. Reeling with negative thoughts about how she would be able to manage to pay her taxes, her mortgage, her car payment, and her living expenses, she arrived at her destination. As she stepped out of the cab, she instantly became sweaty and nauseous and felt a sense of impending doom. Managing one step onto the sidewalk, she felt a sudden ripping upper-back pain that totally consumed her. She fell to the ground, unconscious.

Natalie was rushed to the hospital in cardiac arrest, where her arrival was eagerly anticipated by fifteen hospital staff, two cardiologists, and an emergency room physician. As her gurney burst through the door escorted by four paramedics, advanced cardiac life support was initiated, but despite ninety minutes of aggressive and exhaustive efforts to keep her alive, Natalie tragically passed away. The feeling of defeat in the emergency room was palpable.

After a family meeting with the doctors and the hospital chaplain, the family requested an autopsy, which revealed a ruptured aortic aneurysm as the cause of death. Further testing confirmed the diagnosis of Marfan syndrome.

Cardiologist's Analysis: A Bursting Balloon

Aortic aneurysms are caused by the weakening of the vessel wall, which causes the blood vessel to dilate and makes it prone to bursting like an overfilled balloon. Atherosclerosis (plaque) and high blood pressure both weaken the vessel wall.

Less common causes, as in the case of Natalie, are inherited diseases that are associated with weakened arterial walls. In these diseases, the walls of the arteries are composed of abnormal connective tissue that makes the blood vessels prone to dilate, stretch, and tear. Examples of such diseases are Marfan, Turner's, and Ehlers-Danlos syndromes.

In all these inherited disorders, problems with the connective tissue or the composition of the vessel wall causes progressive weakening and dilation of the ascending aorta—and ultimately, if it's not monitored, aortic rupture. Most patients with dilated aortas are asymptomatic and often don't come in for care until the aorta ruptures. The vast majority of patients with the disease have high blood pressure.

Many people with aortic aneurysms are unaware that the relentless killer is lurking inside them. They cruise through life unaware of their delicate and vulnerable tissue, until suddenly the wall of the fragile aorta tears and gives way. At this point, treatment options are few, and the mortality rate for a ruptured aortic aneurysm exceeds 50 percent. In fact, more than half of all patients who experience the rupture of a thoracic aortic aneurysm die before they reach the hospital. Even more discouraging is that surgical repair of a ruptured thoracic aneurysm is an emergency procedure and carries a 25 to 50 percent mortality rate; when such aneurysms are treated electively, there is only a 5 to 8 percent mortality rate.

The key, as with all disease, is to prevent complications well before any signs or symptoms occur.

Marfan Syndrome and Aortic Rupture

Natalie was diagnosed with an uncommon but known cause of aortic rupture, Marfan syndrome. The diagnosis of Marfan syndrome depends on taking a good family history. It is an inherited disease, so a family history of aortic aneurysm and rupture often, though not always, exists. Natalie's family reported that two cousins on her mother's side of the family died suddenly at young ages. Other similarities included tall stature and unusually long arms and fingers.

Research has shown that the weakened blood vessel walls in Marfan syndrome are caused by a mutation in the gene that plays an important role in the scaffolding of the body's elastic connective tissue. The abnormal connective tissue leads to problems with the aorta, the eyes, and the skin. The patients, like Natalie, are typically tall, with long limbs and spiderlike fingers, chest-wall abnormalities, curvature of the spine, an arched palate, and crowded teeth. All these findings were reported in Natalie's autopsy. Natalie also had recently seen an optometrist and was diagnosed with nearsightedness, a common eye problem seen in Marfan syndrome.

The most common and significant defects in Marfan syndrome are cardiovascular abnormalities such as aortic root enlargement, a leaky aortic valve (aortic regurgitation), and, as in Natalie's case, an aortic aneurysm with a rupture. The most common signs of Marfan syndrome are the following:

- A family history of Marfan syndrome
- A long, lanky frame
- Long, thin limbs
- An arm span that is significantly longer than body height

- Long, spidery fingers
- A thin, narrow face
- Funnel chest or pigeon breast
- Scoliosis
- Visual difficulties
- Flat feet
- Learning disability
- Micrognathia (small lower jaw)
- Coloboma of the iris (a hole in the structure of the eye)
- Hypotonia (deficient muscle tone)

Treatment

Once a diagnosis is made, an annual echocardiography and a chest CT are used to monitor progressive aortic root and ascending aortic dilation. Of all the complications of Marfan syndrome, cardiovascular complications that involve the dilation of the ascending aorta are the most worrisome and potentially life-threatening. The therapeutic goal for affected individuals is to decrease the dilation of the aorta. Medications that decrease the stress on the weakened arterial walls include beta blockers and angiotensin-converting enzyme (ACE) inhibitors. When a family history of Marfan has been discovered or a diagnosis has been made, the individual should avoid anything that could cause undue stress on the delicate arterial system, such as competitive athletics and avoidable stressful situations. In some cases, surgical replacement of the aortic root and valve is necessary.

In a study published in the *American Journal of Cardiology*, thirty-six out of ninety patients with aortic aneurysmal rupture reported experiencing a severe emotional blow in the form of upsetting news: a diagnosis of lung cancer, a big loss at the casino, or having to take a stressful business trip. The study concluded that emotional stress increases blood pressure to the point where the tensile limit of the aortic tissue is overwhelmed, and a rupture occurs. Although Natalie had been weakened by the chronic strain caused by years of competitive athletics, the final blow to her fragile aorta was the emotional stress caused by the alarming news of enormous unpaid taxes. Her tragic outcome gives new meaning to "death and taxes."

If you, a relative, or someone you know has Marfan syndrome, make sure that the person seeks professional consultation. Appropriate counseling can lead to the diagnosis of a medically treatable hereditary condition, in both the affected individual and in family members who may unknowingly be affected.

Our Patient and Family

Natalie's death was felt around the world. Her family was inundated with reams of sympathy cards and piles of elaborate floral arrangements that made it difficult at times to open their front door. Local and national news media covered the tragic loss for weeks and camped outside the home eager to interview Natalie's family. At first, her family was annoyed by the commotion and felt it was an invasion of their privacy. After meeting as a family, though, they agreed that Natalie's wish would be for them to politely oblige. After a few days of interviews they realized the public interest was more an expression of love and compassion for Natalie and her accomplishments rather than an intrusion or an inconvenience. They quickly became versed in the subject and acted as ambassadors for Marfan syndrome, feeling it was their duty to educate the public about this rare and potentially lethal disease.

Just before hearing the horrible news and final confirmation of his sister's death, Natalie's brother Ed noticed a pamphlet that described the B-R-E-A-T-H-E technique conveniently located on a coffee table in the emergency room lobby. A voracious reader and a quick study, Ed learned the technique and taught it to his sisters and brother. To this day, the family attributes their success during this trying time to this helpful, stress-relieving tool. They regularly used the Solid Oak Exercise (reviewed in a later chapter), which helped them relax and cope during this difficult time. It also helped them to understand the importance of knowing your family's medical history and how the B-R-E-A-T-H-E technique is effective in lowering blood pressure, a major treatment for preventing complications of Marfan syndrome.

Running on Empty: Stress and ARVD

Laura Molinari, just seventeen at the time of her cardiac event, is the daughter of first-generation Italian Americans who are living a lifelong dream of economic freedom. Laura's father, Carlos, and her mother, Maria, own a pastry shop in Boston's North End, and every day after school Laura would dutifully walk to the shop and help her parents for several hours.

One day a visitor to the store introduced himself as a modeling agent and persuaded Carlos and Maria to have a professional photographer take a series of pictures of their daughter. He was convinced that Laura had all the makings of a successful model.

Laura had always secretly dreamed of becoming a famous model when she grew up and being able to wear all the clothes she saw in fancy shop windows on Newbury Street in downtown Boston. She was ecstatic when the photo shoot went well and the phone started ringing with offers for local modeling jobs.

Determined to keep her tall, ultra-slim figure and looks, Laura embarked on a secret regimen shared by many other teenage girls. She ate very little, did not drink enough fluids, and worked out physically to an extreme.

One Sunday morning in the spring of 2007, Laura woke late and decided to go on her daily five-mile run before eating or drinking anything. As she passed the three-mile mark, she felt a sudden flutter in her chest and was simultaneously startled by the loud, unexpected gong of the bells of the Cathedral of the Holy Cross. The ear-piercing gong of the cathedral's bells caused a massive flood of adrenaline, and Laura lost consciousness while in midstride.

Fortunately, ten o'clock Mass was just ending, and an exiting flock of churchgoers saw her stumble and fall. They rushed to her side, and one bystander immediately called 911 while another started CPR. The paramedics were on the scene almost immediately, and during the short ride to the nearest hospital, Laura's heart required multiple shocks and advanced cardiac life support (ACLS).

In the emergency room, a cardiologist was consulted, and the ECG that was administered revealed a peculiar and subtle finding known as an epsilon wave. Once Laura's heart rhythm was stabilized, a cardiac MRI was ordered, which revealed fatty tissue density at the tip of her heart. A diagnosis of arrhythmogenic right ventricular dysplasia (ARVD) was made, and a defibrillator was implanted to prevent future events.

Cardiologist's Analysis: The Epsilon Wave, a Subtle Clue

For a diagnosis of ARVD, specific findings on the ECG, the echocardiogram, and the cardiac MRI must be present. Some classic findings that helped to clinch the diagnosis of ARVD in Laura are the following:

- *ECG* A small subtle notch, known as an epsilon wave, was seen. The epsilon wave is found in about 50 percent of those with ARVD.

- *Echocardiography* This revealed an enlarged, weakly contracting right ventricle with a paper-thin wall.

- *Cardiac MRI* Fatty infiltration of the right ventricular wall was visible.

- *Family history* On further questioning, a family history of ARVD and the sudden deaths of three of Laura's Italian relatives were reported.

ARVD: A Family Issue

ARVD is a genetic disease in which the muscle tissue in the lower right chamber of the heart (the right ventricle) is replaced by fat. These fatty patches in the right ventricular muscle can lead to dangerous abnormal heart rhythms (arrhythmias), particularly when a person is under physical or emotional stress.

ARVD is an inherited condition, and patients have a 50 percent chance of passing it on to their children. ARVD is an important cause of ventricular arrhythmias in children and young adults. It's more common in males than females, and in up to 50 percent of cases, another family member is also affected with the disease. As in Laura's case, symptoms usually start in adolescence, are often exercise-related, and commonly occur while competing in athletics. Studies have shown that ARVD is a significant cause of sudden cardiac death among young athletes.

ARVD affects about one in ten thousand people in the general population of the United States, yet some studies have suggested that it may be as common as one in a thousand. It accounts for up to 17 percent of all sudden cardiac deaths in the young.

ARVD is even more common in Italy: it affects forty out of every ten thousand people, making it the most common cause of sudden cardiac death among young Italians.

Like Laura, who lost consciousness at the entrance of a church, about 80 percent of individuals with ARVD are admitted to hospitals after passing out or suffering a sudden cardiac arrest. The other 20 percent frequently complain of palpitations or fluttering in the chest.

Stressors

All stress increases flooding by toxic hormones, which are poorly tolerated with this condition. Common stressors include the following:

- A startled response to a loud, sudden noise such as the gong of a bell or the shout of a coach
- Dehydration
- Sleep deprivation
- Physical exertion

All these stressors trigger the release of stress hormones, which makes the abnormal right ventricle in ARVD more vulnerable to the near-fatal arrhythmia: ventricular fibrillation.

Treatment

Researchers are currently working to develop a gene therapy for ARVD. In the meantime, treatment for ARVD is aimed at controlling the arrhythmias that could lead to a life-threatening cardiac event.

Anti-arrhythmic drugs that quiet the irritable heart muscle have been reported to be effective in suppressing symptomatic arrhythmias in 70–80 percent of patients. Defibrillators are also helpful for treating the potentially life-threatening arrhythmias. Patients like Laura often require a combination of both.

Our Patient

Laura and her family learned much about the genetic inheritance pattern associated with ARVD as well as the adverse affects of emotional stress on the vulnerable heart muscle. They used the Cherry Blossom Exercise, to imagine a perfectly functioning cardiac electrical system, and the Family Tree–Solid Oak Exercise, which helped them to relax, focus, and appreciate their strong family bonds and the importance of each person's cardiovascular health.

Ruminating on the Heart: Stress and Rheumatic Mitral Stenosis

Anju Manilal was born, raised, and educated in Bangalore, India, before immigrating to the United States and founding what eventually became a multibillion-dollar reseller of computer hardware, software, and peripherals.

She founded the business with the modest savings she had accumulated as a consulting software engineer. Anju developed her business with much initiative and effort and little or no assistance, and she reinvested every dollar of profit. The more her business grew, the greater number of workers were required, but the profit margins in her business were dismally small, and she found herself perpetually worried about cash-flow shortages.

Financial worries began consuming Anju, and she constantly feared that the day would come when she wouldn't be able to buy the necessary inventory, make the payroll, cover the increasingly large fixed costs of doing business, and be able to afford health insurance for her workers. She began to lose weight, and her friends and her coworkers made comments about how exhausted she looked. One night, while alone at home, she began having rapid heart palpitations and a severe shortness of breath. Her pounding heart felt as though it were going to leap out of her chest. She sat alone in tears, wracked by fear, knowing that her worst nightmare was happening: her health was failing her, and if that happened, she would eventually fail the many hundreds of people who had come to count on her.

While Anju was still a young girl in India, a school nurse had told her that she had a heart murmur. Anju had never pursued it, but she always worried that it might surface someday. Now that day had come. Anju recalled how as a child she had been hospitalized in a small village for a sore throat, a severe fever, joint aches, and a peculiar skin rash. Her diagnosis was rheumatic fever, a disorder caused by a streptococcal infection that typically starts with a sore throat.

As Anju's palpitations grew stronger, her breathing became more labored and she felt as though she were drowning, so she desperately grabbed the phone and called 911. The paramedics brought her to the hospital emergency room, where a chest X-ray revealed congestive heart failure and an ECG atrial fibrillation.

Cardiologist's Analysis: Strep Throat, a Tricky Imposter

An echocardiogram revealed that Anju also had severe rheumatic mitral stenosis. A throat infection caused by a common bacterium had tricked her immune system into thinking that the heart valve tissue was the source of the infection. In time, chronic inflammation caused thickening and decreased mobility of her mitral valve, which connects the upper left chamber (the left atrium) with the lower left chamber (the left ventricle).

There are a few classic findings that a cardiologist hears when listening to a patient with mitral stenosis. Because the valve doors are thickened and tethered together from chronic inflammation, both the opening and the closing of the valve are accentuated. The closing is loud because of increased force created by pressure between the left atrium and the left ventricle. A heart murmur is created from blood flowing from the top chamber to the bottom chamber through a narrowed opening.

Other signs of rheumatic mitral stenosis in a physical exam are rosy cheeks, swollen ankles, and an irregular pulse due to atrial fibrillation. The most common symptom of mitral stenosis, seen in about 70 percent of patients, is shortness of breath.

Because Anju had severe shortness of breath even while she was at rest, her cardiologist believed that she would require more than medication to treat her valve problem. She was thought to be a good candidate for either balloon valvuloplasty or mitral valve replacement. She opted for the former.

The Cause of Rheumatic Mitral Stenosis

In rheumatic mitral stenosis, the valve doors become thickened and fail to open properly because of chronic inflammation, which is caused by a streptococcus infection. The saloonlike doors lose their mobility and become permanently stuck in one position, as if they had severely rusted hinges. The flow of blood from the left atrium to the left ventricle is impeded, and the subsequent buildup of blood in the upper chamber of the heart backs up into the lungs, which causes various degrees of shortness of breath, or *dyspnea*.

The congestion or backup of blood in rheumatric mitral stenosis is worsened when the heart rate increases, because this causes a decrease in the amount of time it takes for blood to empty into the bottom chamber. This causes more and more congestion and hence more difficulty breathing.

Rheumatic fever, a major cause of mitral stenosis, has been nearly eradicated in the United States due to the wide availability of antibiotics. In countries where antibiotics are less readily available, however, it still exists. In some developing countries, such as India, the prevalence of rheumatic fever is 100 to 150 cases per 100,000 people. Anju vividly recalled her childhood episode of rheumatic fever that was the cause of her mitral stenosis. She had had a fever, a sore throat, a rash, and arthritis, which are classic in rheumatic fever. Years later she developed a heart murmur and symptoms.

The evolution of the development of mitral stenosis from rheumatic fever, as in Anju's case, is a phase with no symptoms followed by shortness of breath and palpitations. The average asymptomatic latent period is more than sixteen years. Once the symptoms of mitral stenosis begin to develop, the progression to severe disability can take an additional decade.

Stressors

Exercise, emotional stress, pregnancy, infection, and fever can increase the heart rate and make the symptoms of mitral stenosis worse. Increased amounts of toxic stress hormones are poorly tolerated in this condition. The triggers of Anju's symptoms included the following:

- Emotional stress (work stress and financial worries)
- Dehydration
- Sleep deprivation
- Viral bronchitis leading to lower blood oxygen levels
- Fever

All these stressors lead to a surge of stress hormones and an increased heart rate, which is particularly poorly tolerated in the context of mitral stenosis. A higher heart rate decreases the amount of time that the left ventricle has to fill up, which causes the backup or congestion of blood in the lungs due to the blocked mitral valve.

Treatment

Treatment options for mitral stenosis include the following:

- Medical management with drugs that slow the heart rate to improve the filling of the left ventricle, such as beta blockers and calcium channel blockers
- Surgical replacement of the valve
- Percutaneous balloon valvuloplasty (opening a constricted heart valve using a balloon threaded through the blood vessels)

To determine which patients would benefit from percutaneous balloon valvuloplasty, a scoring system has been developed that is based on four echocardiographic criteria:

1. Valve door mobility
2. Valve door thickening
3. Subvalvar thickening
4. Calcification

Early on, treatment for mitral stenosis involves medications that slow the heart and optimize filling to promote forward blood flow. As the disease advances, the hinges on the valve doors become rusty and the movement of the movement is progressively restricted. Eventually mechanical therapies including balloon valvuloplasty and valve replacement are required to relieve the obstruction.

Our Patient

During the postoperative recovery period, Anju used the Boulders Exercise to imagine a perfectly functioning mitral valve and a freely flowing cardiac system. This helped to expedite her recovery so that she could return to work.

Several years later, Anju is still running a successful business. She also provides a healthy work environment for her employees by offering healthy food choices in the cafeteria, weekly yoga and massage sessions, and the B-R-E-A-T-H-E technique.

Stress: Horses and Zebras Drink from the Same Trough

What is shared by both common and uncommon cardiac conditions is *stress* and the negative impact that a surge of stress hormones can have on the various heart parts. Adrenaline and cortisol can lead to devastating cardiovascular complications.

Another similarity shared by common and uncommon cardiac conditions is the beneficial effect of the B-R-E-A-T-H-E technique. It stimulates the relaxation response, blunts the release of stress hormones, and helps the heart to work more efficiently.

Some of the conditions discussed in this chapter are rare but may seem vaguely familiar because celebrity involvement has led to media coverage, increased public interest, and increased education. Professional basketball players, news commentators, Olympic athletes, and supermodels are among those who have been afflicted by these rare disorders and have helped to heighten public awareness.

Two of the four conditions discussed here have a strong genetic link, so family members should be particularly aware of the negative effects of stress and the positive effects that B-R-E-A-T-H-E can have on their hearts, too.

11

Heart-Warming Stories

You've learned how the B-R-E-A-T-H-E technique can help to strengthen the hearts of patients with specific heart conditions, soothe the hearts of compassionate caregivers and supportive family members, and provide an effective escape route from the powerful jaws of sudden stress.

Now you'll learn another application for this simple and helpful technique: you'll see how people faced with adversity have not only changed their lives for the better but have also used the B-R-E-A-T-H-E technique as a trusty rudder with which to navigate rough waters and as an anchor when the waters are calm. You'll learn how committing to a regular daily practice will help you to maintain an excellent quality of life.

In the following stories, you'll see how B-R-E-A-T-H-E inspired new beginnings and provided a breath of fresh air for those who were faced with adversity and hardship. As you read the stories, apply what you've learned about the B-R-E-A-T-H-E technique to the challenges each person faced; identify the various triggers of stress, the bodily cues that resulted from the conversation, and how each affected individual incorporated B-R-E-A-T-H-E into his or her busy lives.

The B-R-E-A-T-H-E technique can fit into even the most harried and demanding schedule. It helps people to effectively manage stress, experience improved sleep, enhance their mental focus, and achieve their life goals.

Under the Gun

Bob Jefferson worked for the Illinois Department of Corrections as a parole officer for twenty-nine years. Promoted multiple times throughout his career, he was eventually placed in charge of a hundred plainclothes officers, and their job was to arrest parolees who had violated their parole.

The work involved in bringing these individuals to justice often required tremendous physical and mental fortitude. Pursuits frequently ended in physical and violent scuffles, and throughout the years, the many altercations had even led to death threats against Bob and his family.

At fifty-nine, he knew that his endurance was running out, and he was really beginning to feel the pace of his emotionally charged job. In the past year, two of his most loyal and dedicated parole officers had succumbed to the tremendous pressure of the job and committed suicide.

Bob's biggest worry was for his safety and that of the people who reported to him. Their assignments often involved going into housing projects, where violence was commonplace. The people in the neighborhoods began to recognize him when he entered their neighborhood, and within moments signals were sent from house to house notifying others of his arrival. This made the job of locating parolees even more difficult.

Bob grew paranoid and worried that people knew who he was. Although he didn't wear a uniform, he was assumed to be a potential threat to the community and viewed by most of the neighborhoods as someone with a gun and the power to handcuff and arrest.

One day, while Bob was at the firing range, he had a breakdown after repeatedly struggling to pull his gun from his concealed holster and then performing miserably on the target practice. He realized he'd been kidding himself: he could no longer protect himself or his loyal employees. In the nights that followed, he had repetitive nightmares about a parolee wrestling him to the ground, getting control of his gun, and shooting him.

Finally, after the most stressful year of his career, Bob retired. During the first three months, he had difficulty letting go of the job and frequently visited the office to consult with new recruits and help them with the intricacies of the job. Eventually, with the strong urging of his wife and his children, he completely removed himself from the corrections office and found a sense of peace in completely "washing his hands" of the stressful job.

The first year of Bob's retirement turned out to be difficult and filled with a number of heart-related health issues. He thought that all the years of emotional stress had finally caught up with him, and it seemed ironic that the proverbial wheels had started falling off the wagon only once he had retired.

Bob began experiencing daily chest pain when he walked his dog. He even started becoming anxiety-ridden and paranoid when his neighbors greeted him, believing that they saw him as "the parole officer." His chest pain became more frequent and severe. Finally, one day after he had walked his dog, the pain felt like an elephant on his chest, so he called 911.

Cardiologist's Analysis: Heal with Steel

Bob was taken to the emergency room, where he was met by a cardiologist and immediately given a coronary angiogram. This revealed 90 percent blockages in each of his three major coronary arteries, and bypass surgery was recommended to repair it.

Sometimes, when coronary artery disease is extensive, as in Bob's case, coronary bypass surgery is indicated. In reference to the stainless steel scalpel used by the surgeon, cardiologists ask that the cardiovascular surgeons "heal with steel."

Despite his trepidation, Bob cruised through the surgery. He had a minor postoperative event on the fourth day, when he developed a slow heart rate. This required the implantation of a pacemaker to keep his heart rate steady. Seven days after surgery, he was discharged in stable condition.

B-R-E-A-T-H-E
Bypassing the Blockage

One year, three hospitalizations, a triple bypass surgery, and a pacemaker later, Bob began practicing the B-R-E-A-T-H-E techniques. His favorites are the River Exercise and the Cherry Blossom Exercise, which help him to concentrate on improved blood flow and his heart's electrical current after his bypass and pacemaker surgeries.

During his daily practice, Bob broadens the focus of his exercise and spends time concentrating on his passion for teaching and mentoring troubled youth at Lawson's YMCA in Chicago.

Burned Out on Bereavement

Spencer O'Malley was a New York City fireman for twenty-five years. He loved his job more than anything on the planet, but his world changed dramatically on 9/11, when his partner of more than twenty years died in the World Trade Center.

While the second tower was still barely standing, Spencer and his partner and lifelong friend, Dave Reilly, decided to make one final run into the smoke created by the debris of molten steel and ash; their mission was to rescue people trapped on the ground level of the disaster zone. As they prepared to enter the barely recognizable structure, Spencer gave Dave one final nod as they entered the building. Suddenly a massive steel post fell. This is the last thing that Spencer remembers happening until someone placed an oxygen mask on his face to revive him. His partner and best friend didn't make it out of the building.

In the next three weeks Spencer attended twenty funerals for fallen friends and coworkers. Then he was asked by Dave's family to do the eulogy for his partner. Though physically and emotionally exhausted, he agreed.

As Spencer read aloud the eulogy he had written, he didn't think he would make it to completion. As he struggled through his sobs to tell the story of how he and Dave had met in the third grade and promised each other that one day they'd be firemen with the New York Fire Department, he became aware that he was having trouble catching his breath. He wasn't sure whether it was due to the emotionally charged event or to something else.

After the heartfelt eulogy, family and friends surrounded him at the podium. He suddenly began gasping for air, excused himself, and ran out of the church. Once outside, he finally seemed to be able to catch his breath.

Spencer attributed his breathing problem to his nerves, but his symptoms persisted. He had trouble walking less than a block from the church to his car and had to stop multiple times to catch his breath. Once he had a horrible night; he was unable to sleep and had to get up hourly to urinate. At one point he ran to the bedroom window and frantically flung it open to get some fresh air. Finally, at four o'clock in the morning, he fell into an unsettled sleep after propping his head up on four pillows. Waking up short of breath, Spencer called his doctor, who instructed him to get to the hospital immediately.

Cardiologist's Analysis: The Heart Unloaded

Spencer's symptoms of severe sudden shortness of breath were from congestive heart failure. The symptoms of congestive heart failure progress from mild shortness of breath with exertion to severe shortness of breath at rest. The mildest form is characterized by shortness of breath after climbing two flights of stairs carrying two bags of groceries.

Spencer has the most severe form, with symptoms occurring at rest. His symptoms worsen when he lies down, because gravity forces fluid into his lungs, which compromises the flow of oxygen and leads to shortness of breath. Here are some facts about the condition:

- The symptom of shortness of breath when lying down is known as *orthopnea*. It implies a failing heart and congestion.

- A severe form of orthopnea is paroxysmal nocturnal dyspnea (PND), in which patients suddenly get out of bed to catch their breath.

- To prevent orthopnea from occurring and to be able to fall asleep, patients often innately know to either sleep in a sitting position or prop themselves up with multiple pillows.

- Frequent urination during the night is a telltale sign of congestion and is known as *nocturia*. Nocturia occurs because of the following: As the body struggles to maintain blood flow to the brain during the day, the kidneys are relatively deprived of blood flow. At night, when the body is less active, the kidneys are supplied with more flow, leading to increased urination.

The cardiologist ordered three tests (a chest X-ray, an echocardiogram, and a special blood test known as a BNP, or brain naturietic peptide), and they clinched the diagnosis of congestive heart failure. Spencer's chest X-ray revealed an enlarged heart and fluid in his lungs. His BNP was elevated, which confirmed that his heart pump was overloaded with fluid. His echocardiogram showed a severely weakened pump.

The presumable cause of the severe muscle damage to Spencer's heart was long-standing high blood pressure, which Spencer had struggled with throughout his life.

He was started on a number of medicines, including an ACE inhibitor, a diuretic, and a beta blocker. These drugs serve to maximize the efficiency of the heart by optimizing the "loading of the heart," which refers to how volume (preload) and pressure (afterload) affect the function of the heart. In patients with congestive heart failure, preload, or volume, tends to be excessive and is manifested clinically by signs of swelling in the arms, legs, and even face; fluid backing up into the lungs causes varying degrees of shortness of breath. "Afterload" refers to the pressure and force required by the main pump (left ventricle) to propel blood forward to the body.

Diuretics remove fluid and reduce preload, and ACE inhibitors dilate arteries, lowering pressure, or afterload. Beta blockers block the effects of the stress hormone adrenaline, which also has an afterload-reducing effect. Both interventions make it easier for the weakened heart muscle to pump blood forward.

Within two weeks he was able to walk five miles at a brisk pace and sleep lying down through the night without interruption.

B-R-E-A-T-H-E
A Fresh Start

While he was in the hospital, Spencer had a lot of time to think. He had enough years of service to be able to retire, but he felt torn between giving up his lifelong passion and slowing down in order to spend more quality time with his wife. His retirement would end a legacy of firefighters in his family, and he felt obligated to follow in the footsteps of his father and his grandfather and finish thirty years with the department.

Spencer knew that firefighting was taking a toll on his health, however, and he had read that 50 percent of the firemen who had died in the previous year in the line of duty had had heart attacks. He also knew that studies have shown that firefighters have elevated heart rates while in the line of duty for prolonged periods, thereby putting undue stress on their hearts. Finally, after a lot of careful thought and in the interest of his health, Spencer decided to retire.

Spencer began using the B-R-E-A-T-H-E technique to focus, relax, and heal his heart. Before his four-mile morning walk, he began regularly practicing the Fallen Tree Exercise and the Path of Relaxation Exercise.

One day, during his focused relaxation session, Spencer found himself thinking about trains. Both he and Dave had been train buffs since childhood, and he recalled the two of them walking the train tracks near their homes in the Bronx and fantasizing that one day they'd travel on trains all the way to the West Coast.

During the next few weeks, while he was doing his B-R-E-A-T-H-E exercises, he found himself recalling that some of the most tranquil times in his life were when he would sit on his back porch and listen to the sounds of the trains passing by before he went to bed.

Spencer and his wife, Jeanine, decided to make a fresh start and move to California, where he got a job with Amtrak as a train conductor. At each stop along the ride up and down the California coast, he collects all the tickets and then retires to the conductor's seat, where he practices his B-R-E-A-T-H-E technique, calmly envisioning his heart as strong and powerful like the river in his exercises and the train on which he rides.

Healthy Workplace, Healthy Business

Since the third grade at prep school in New England, Simon Barrington had always been first in his class. He graduated summa cum laude from Columbia University, which guaranteed him a spot at his next destination of choice, Harvard Business School. There he quickly gained a reputation as a whiz kid who sat in the front row of every class and had the answers ready before the professor asked the questions.

Simon's Ivy League connections and his fierce ultra-competitive nature helped him to land his first job at a venture capital firm in Silicon Valley. As usual, within months he had advanced far beyond the other new hires, and he began his ascension to the top ranks. After only two years, but with a few million dollars more to his name, he quit the firm, teamed up with two friends from Harvard, and started a software company.

Their novel idea for business software that would organize stock portfolios and signal buying and selling opportunities was quickly recognized as the best idea in years by top executives at the largest brokerage house on Wall Street. This brokerage firm was going to make a huge investment in Simon's company; then, just weeks before, a huge fight erupted over how the eventual stock would be divided, and one partner and five of the fledging firm's ten staff members walked out. In their absence, Simon and the remaining partner and staffers began pulling all-nighters and catching an occasional hour or two of sleep in the office. Simon promised his wife that the moment the deal was done, he'd be there for her and their newborn son.

Simon and his team flew off to New York to sign the papers and celebrate, but while waiting to shake the final hand in the mahogany-walled boardroom, Simon felt as though his heart had jumped out of his body. He became nauseous and so light-headed that he almost passed out, and he was rushed to New York–Presbyterian Hospital.

In the emergency room, the doctor quickly evaluated Simon's palpitations, light-headedness, and sweating as a prodrome (a set of symptoms associated with arrhythmia just before passing out) and ordered an ECG, which revealed a heart rate of two hundred beats per minute. The doctor immediately began an intravenous administration of adenosine, which quickly slowed Simon's rapid heart rate and quieted his arrhythmia. The doctor then ordered a consultation with a cardiologist.

Cardiologist's Analysis: Removing the Irritable Spot

After hearing Simon's story, performing a physical exam, and reviewing his ECG, the cardiologist diagnosed atrioventricular nodal reentry tachycardia (AVNRT). He explained that Simon had a tiny "ticklish" spot in his cardiac electrical system that was triggered by an excess of adrenaline in his bloodstream.

He added that lack of sleep, caffeine, and dehydration all contributed to the event. Simon was discharged after being scheduled for an elective procedure known as radio frequency (RF) ablation.

This procedure involved passing a small catheter up through his right groin and removing the "ticklish" tissue by emitting RF waves and heat at the location of the paroxysmal supraventricular tachycardia (PSVT). At the end of the procedure, Simon was brought to the recovery room, where his wife and infant son were waiting anxiously. As the cardiologist discussed the success of the procedure, Simon's wife gave him a huge hug and a kiss while they held their son in their arms.

B-R-E-A-T-H-E
Healthy Software

Soon after his successful procedure, Simon began using the B-R-E-A-T-H-E exercises. During his meditations he came to realize that he had placed the achievement of success far ahead of his family and his friends. Upon realizing that love and time with family is priceless, he decided to change both the name and the direction of his company. He renamed it Namaste (an Indian greeting that means "I bow to the divine goodness in you") and began to develop a very different kind of software, named Prana (the Sanskrit term for the life-breath connection). Now, instead of allowing every deal to become a personal life-or-death struggle, Simon spends much of his time designing programs to reward his employees and his clients for becoming interested in their health and well-being. The company awards bonuses for exercising, eating a healthy diet, and practicing relaxation skills such as yoga, tai chi, and B-R-E-A-T-H-E.

Greening with Envy

John Dixon is the CEO of Green Earth Life, a company that builds and manages health spas for hotels, resorts, and cruise ships around the world. Ironically, John—who spent more than two hundred nights a year on the road scouting out new opportunities, closing deals, and solving the day-to-day problems of running a business— never used any of the relaxation services his spas offer.

One day, John, who had a well-known reputation for never slowing down and relaxing, was standing at the end of a conference table urging a group of hotel executives to let his company take over the management of their hotel's spas when he suddenly collapsed. However, he quickly regained consciousness and said he felt fine.

Cardiologist's Analysis: Not Necessary

John never actually saw a cardiologist. An on-site nurse practitioner performed an ECG, which revealed rapid atrial fibrillation. His blood oxygen level was less than 90 percent, so the nurse-practitioner began administering oxygen and called for an ambulance.

In the hospital John was administered medication to slow down his rapid heartbeat and was given an echocardiogram, which showed normal heart function and normal heart valves. Lab tests showed that he was dehydrated, and tests to rule out a heart attack or thyroid problems were both negative. He was given a one-liter dose of intravenous saline fluid and discharged.

When he returned home from his business trip, John went straight to his general internist, who ordered a treadmill test to rule out blocked arteries. The test results were normal. After ruling out all possible structural heart problems, his doctor concluded that the emotional stress created by the pressure of performing in front of an audience of potential investors triggered the event. The doctor suggested that dehydration and sleeping poorly from jet lag had contributed to increased levels of stress hormones.

B – R – E – A – T – H – E

From Selling Relaxation to Experiencing It

A friend told John about the B-R-E-A-T-H-E exercises, and he began doing them regularly. His favorite exercise is the Path of Relaxation, which he uses every morning and before every presentation. Another relaxation ploy that helps him to focus is to begin each presentation with a story that describes in detail the wonderful journey that will be taken if the people he's talking to decide to work with his company. Practicing what he had been preaching (or rather, selling) made the business journey much more pleasurable for John, and the B-R-E-A-T-H-E exercises have helped him to remain relaxed and keep his presentations entertaining, engaging, and sharp.

Flooded

New Orleans resident Caroline Sherman is a story of success against all odds. Born to a fourteen-year-old mother and raised by a series of relatives whose homes were frequently filled with domestic violence, drugs, and alcoholism, she was determined to provide a better life for her four-year-son, Jami.

Her life had been a huge struggle and had taken its toll, but she had managed to graduate with honors from Tulane University. She had a great job in human resources with a Fortune 500 company and was working at night on an MBA.

Although Caroline's accomplishment-filled life looked good from the outside, there was constant stress on the inside. Because of the costs of child care, tuition and books, a car payment, and rent that seemed to increase every few months, money was always tight. From time to time Caroline would feel overwhelmed and notice heart palpitations and shortness of breath. During one particularly stressful time, she visited a local emergency room, where a rather snippy young doctor told her that she was only suffering from anxiety and wrote up a prescription for Xanax, a commonly prescribed antianxiety medicine. Despite what the doctor said were normal ECG and lab test results, Caroline's intuition told her that something was going on that wasn't right.

Caroline went home and got on the Internet, and what she found was disturbing. Women tend to have vastly different symptoms for heart disease than men do, the condition is routinely misdiagnosed in women, and frequently they're shunted aside by doctors as just being anxiety-ridden.

Cardiologist's Analysis: Stents Help Weather the Storm

Caroline immediately arranged a consultation with a New Orleans cardiologist, who performed a stress test, diagnosed multiple blocked arteries, and subsequently stented two major blood vessels. When she was moved from the ICU into a regular hospital room, Caroline telephoned who her mother, who was caring for her son, and told her that everything went well and that she'd be home the following day. That night, as she lay in her hospital bed with her heart problems resolved, she thought about her life and the fact that she could do and have it all.

The next day, shortly after she arrived home, Hurricane Katrina hit New Orleans. She frantically called her mother and received no answer. She finally reached a neighbor of her mother's who told her that everyone on the block had been evacuated to the Superdome. Caroline managed to get to the Superdome, and after hours of frantic searching, she found her mother and her son. Katrina destroyed her home and her mother's home, but in the months that followed the disaster, Caroline kept taking deep breaths, handling things one step at a time, and promising herself that she would make everything work.

B-R-E-A-T-H-E
Hurricane and Heart Healing

A friend introduced Caroline to the B-R-E-A-T-H-E technique, which she credits with getting her through the rough times that every resident of New Orleans faced. The B-R-E-A-T-H-E exercises allowed Caroline to reassess her life. Her favorite exercises are the River Exercise and the Path of Relaxation. As Caroline learned how to deal with stress by breathing and relaxing, she began to see clearly what she wanted in her life. She eventually built a business plan for a day-care center for working mothers that utilized all her talents. Within a year after Katrina, Caroline had not just a heart that had been repaired and was healthy but also a booming day-care center, a new home, and a fulfilled life. She credits B-R-E-A-T-H-E with giving her and Jami the life she had dreamed of having.

Stress, Traffic, and the Heart

Julie Meriweather, a retired aerospace engineer, spent most of her time with two young grandchildren, Owen and Andy, rambunctious identical twins who gave new meaning to the term *terrible twos*. What with grocery shopping, tandem stroller rides in the park, and seemingly endless diaper changes, Julie had little time for herself, but she believed it was her duty to help her single daughter, Cindy, watch the kids while Cindy worked as a checkout person at the local market.

Julie was already overextending herself, but she managed to squeeze in a visit to her doctor. This was just a regular checkup, but she did talk to her doctor about her family history of colon cancer. She was promptly scheduled for a colonoscopy, a procedure she had been dreading for years, but now the day had come for her to face the reality and be screened. Her reluctance to undergo the procedure was created partly by her fear of being diagnosed with cancer, like so many of her relatives, but also because she had a dreadful fear of needles (the required shots of antianxiety and sedative medications for the procedure).

After her doctor carefully explained the indications, the risks, and the potential complications of the procedure, Julie began to worry frantically about it all. She actually started to sweat whenever the thought of the needle crossed her mind.

The day finally arrived. She left the kids with her daughter and had a neighbor ride with her to the hospital. They left early, as her doctor suggested, so that she would have plenty of time to park and not be late. Unfortunately once they got on the interstate highway, they encountered unexpected major traffic. The highway looked like a parking lot, and the five-lane, winding queue of cars seemed to go on for miles.

Julie and her neighbor realized that they were locked in, with cars in front, behind, and on both sides. They were enmeshed in this painfully sluggish route, unable to exit. Julie quickly found the local traffic station on the radio, which reported that a large diesel truck had overturned and spilled petroleum all over the highway, causing traffic to back up for fifty miles. The news reporter told commuters to be prepared for major delays due to the highway being "all clogged up."

Once traffic began to move again at a snail's pace, Julie was already forty-five minutes late. The more she glanced at her watch, the more nervous she became, and when she finally exited the highway she was a nervous wreck. She began to drive recklessly down side streets, honking needlessly at cars in front of her on her way to the hospital.

Her neighbor held on for dear life as Julie sped down crowded city streets. Despite her neighbor's repeated polite requests, Julie refused to slow down. Once she arrived at the hospital, she literally skidded to a stop at the hospital entrance; with the car still running, Julie jumped out and barked at her neighbor to park the car.

As Julie approached the hospital admissions desk, she felt her heart racing and had trouble catching her breath. The medical receptionist at the desk noticed that she was having trouble completing sentences and quickly consulted a nearby nurse, who promptly grabbed a wheelchair and whisked Julie to the preoperative area. There she met her gastroenterologist, who was understanding about her tardiness because of the uncontrollable traffic and told her not to worry.

Yet worry Julie did. As if traffic hadn't been bad enough, the next step—the dreaded needle—made her go ballistic. As her doctor explained the procedure again to her, the nurse began to prep her arm for the IV, and just as the doctor asked her to sign the consent form, her mind became a blur and her heart began to race. The heart monitor registered her heart rate at more than two hundred beats per minute and her blood pressure at 200/90. This led the doctor to cancel the procedure and schedule a cardiology consultation.

Cardiologist's Analysis: All Clogged Up

Julie's story represents two common stressful triggers that I commonly see in my practice: congested traffic and the anxiety created by an anticipated surgical procedure.

When I arrived, Julie looked anxious, and beads of sweat had begun to appear on her forehead. Her heart had slowed a bit once she was told that her colonoscopy would be postponed. After I introduced myself, Julie immediately began blaming the horrible traffic for all her symptoms. When she finished her story, I empathized with her and told her that this is a common scenario and that stress from congested traffic has indeed been linked to heart attacks.

She seemed surprised to hear this; then she was relieved that something could account for her rapid heartbeat, shortness of breath, and light-headedness. She said that she had frequently experienced these feelings when she was still working and commuting every day in heavy traffic. The same symptoms would occur when she was stuck in traffic and was late for work. She recalled feeling a sense of panic, which led to palpitations and shortness of breath.

In a German study, patients who had heart attacks were found to be three times as likely to have been in traffic within an hour of the onset of their heart attacks. Although riding public transportation and riding a bicycle were also associated with increased risk, driving a car was the most common type of traffic exposure in those who suffered heart attacks. Overall, being in or on any mode of transportation in traffic was associated with a 3.2 times higher risk than not being in traffic. Those who were affected most by traffic were women, elderly males, patients who were unemployed, and those with a history of angina.

Another phenomenon related to heavy traffic, heart disease, and stress is road rage. Road rage is characterized by sudden, abrupt, and sometimes violent acts of hostility and anger brought about while driving—especially in heavy traffic. The official psychiatric term for road rage is intermittent explosive disorder (IED), and it has been reported to be surprisingly common, occurring in at least 5 percent of the U.S. population.

As you might expect, anger and hostility take a major toll on the heart. In one study, men with high hostility were 1.6 times more likely to die from coronary artery disease than their more placid peers. Researchers in Nova Scotia found that hostility more than doubled the risk of recurrent heart attacks in men—but not in women. Other studies have linked hostility to an increased prevalence of cardiac risk factors, to decreased survival in men with coronary artery disease below the age of sixty-one, to an increased risk of heart attack in men with metabolic syndrome, and to an increased risk of abnormal heart rhythms. To make matters worse, hostility often coexists with depression, which is a cardiac risk factor in and of itself.

Thus, as you can see, if you become stressed, angry, or frustrated while you are driving, you are not alone. Data clearly show a link between heavy traffic and cardiac disease, and whether you're worried about being late or are experiencing road rage, the same stress hormones are surging, causing damage to delicate cardiac tissue.

B-R-E-A-T-H-E

The Fork in the River Exercise

Many of us travel long distances and battle traffic to get to work each day. This can make us feel exhausted even before we get to work. The following exercise is recommended for those who have a heavy daily commute.

This exercise is helpful for reminding us to listen to the heart-brain conversation in the midst of this unavoidable situation. Memorize the images in this exercise and recall them when your commute seems endless. *Do not do this exercise while driving.* When you are not driving, practicing this exercise will help you to remember to listen to the conversation when you're frustrated, then to recall the images that are outlined in the exercise, and finally to associate them with feelings of calm and peace. For best results, practice this exercise in the morning, before you start your daily commute.

Begin

Begin your exercise in your warm, cozy, and familiar place. Wear loose-fitting clothing and settle comfortably in your favorite chair or sofa. Always start your exercise by listening to the conversation. Remember that your heart and your brain are connected and in constant communication. Listen to your heart.

Take a deep breath in through your nose and let it out through your mouth. Count s-l-o-w-l-y to seven. Notice that when you take in a deep breath, your heart rate slightly increases, and as you exhale, your heart rate decreases. Take a few more breaths and notice this trend: in, your heart rate increases; out, your heart rate decreases. The more you practice, the better you will get at hearing your heartbeat. This is excellent proof that you are participating in the conversation.

As you begin, focus on your heart and clear your mind of any other thoughts. Liken this exercise to working out different muscles in the gym. Instead of working your back, your shoulders, or your biceps, look at this exercise as exercising and developing your heart-brain connection.

Relax

Remember that the relaxation response is a state of deep relaxation that is the opposite of the fight-or-flight response. You can reach this state by deep breathing. It is comfortable, sooth-ing, and nurturing for your heart. Breathing in and out causes changes in the heart rate. When you take a deep breath in, you are activating the sympathetic nervous system, which causes your heart rate to speed up. When you exhale, count to seven, like the number of letters in B-R-E-A-T-H-E. This extended exha-lation activates the parasympathetic nervous system and slows the heart rate by sending signals from your brain to your heart on a highway called the vagus nerve. This fluctuation or variabil-ity of the heart rate is good for the heart.

Envision

Gaze down a majestic river, away from a waterfall, and see a fork in the river. Notice the river branching into two separate pathways. One is small, tortuous, and barely flowing. The other is wide, powerful, and flowing rapidly. Notice that as the river branches, the majority of the flow is directed toward the path of least resistance. The larger, more rapid, and free-flowing tribu-tary is lined with lush vegetation and wildlife, whereas the edge of the small, tortuous rivulet is dry and uninhabited. Imagine that the flow of the larger branch is constant and maintained by the strength and force of the waterfall. Notice that the water level of the river is maintained and constant, like your heart in perfect balance.

Apply

Make a mental connection and apply how the fork in the river represents your choice of how to react when you are stuck in traffic. When you are frustrated, imagine how anger and hostility lead to an outpouring of stress hormones, decreasing the blood flow to your tissues, and resemble the small rivulet at the fork in the river whose edges are barren and thirsting for nourishment. You realize that the traffic is unavoidable and that reacting with anger is harmful and unproductive, so instead you imagine that the large branching tributary at the fork in the river is like flowing down the path of least resistance. Imagine that the larger tributary is smooth and unobstructed, like your blood vessels. Note how the beautiful vegetation around you represents your healthy heart. Listen to the sounds around you. The gentle breeze blowing in the trees, the chirping of the birds, and the sound of the distant waterfall all resemble your heart: constant, rhythmic, and powerful.

Treat

View this exercise as a special treatment for yourself. You are deserving of this pleasurable and therapeutic time. The exercise is pleasurable, relaxing, and rejuvenating. This is not a chore or a task. Before long you will look forward to this work and feel like a runner who experiences a high from running.

Remember that this exercise, when performed correctly, is therapeutic and serves to decrease your heart rate, lower your blood pressure, and lower your vascular tone. The deeper and more relaxed you become, the more protective and effective is the therapy. Meditation and exercises such as the B-R-E-A-T-H-E technique are therapeutic: they lower the levels of cardiotoxic hormones such as cortisol and adrenaline. This exercise increases heart-rate variability and low fluctuations in heart rate (low heart-rate variability) in patients who have been diagnosed with poor cardiovascular outcomes. Recall that guided imagery bolsters the immune system, lowers blood pressure and heart rate, and decreases anxiety.

Heal

When using the B-R-E-A-T-H-E technique, imagine the healing properties of relaxation. Your deep breathing helps you to train the nerves that connect the brain and the heart and has a calming and slowing effect on your heart rate. This exercise will reduce stress and make you feel better, which will enhance healing in your body. It will allow you to downshift so that your engine can cool and idle for a while. Imagine that the warm sun on your shoulders causes your blood vessels to dilate, further improving flow and thus healing your electrical system. Store the heart-healing metaphors in your memory so they can be quickly retrieved to help protect and heal your heart when you're stuck in traffic or you're having a difficult commute.

End

As you end your B-R-E-A-T-H-E exercise, recall all of the heart-healing metaphors and summarize their significance and their relationship to your healing heart. Remember the perfectly flowing river and the powerful waterfall. As you end your exercise, you will become aware of your surroundings and feel energized. Your heart is strong, rhythmic, and unobstructed like the river.

Going Under, Not Over

Perhaps the most common stressful trigger I've observed in my patients is the anxiety and fear they experience before a planned surgical procedure. I often tell my patients to be careful not to go *over*board just when they are about to go *under*. Julie is a classic example of this phenomenon. The combination of worrying about her possible diagnosis, being afraid of needles, and arriving late for her procedure caused her to spin out of control. She became so anxious that she wound up with a rapid arrhythmia and her procedure postponed.

People who are undergoing surgical procedures are understandably scared and anxious. The two most common fears are the possibility of a complication or of not waking up from the anesthesia. These feelings and concerns are real and should be thoroughly discussed before surgery with the operating physician. Having a thorough understanding of the procedure and trust in the operating physician is paramount for a healing, successful surgery. When this trust isn't developed, or when people feel uninformed, they become stressed out—and for good reason.

B-R-E-A-T-H-E
The Healing Path of Flow Exercise

At some point in our lives, most of us will either personally experience a surgical procedure or know someone who does. Surgery can be scary and anxiety-provoking.

The following exercise is designed to help those who are undergoing elective surgery relax and feel a sense of calm prior to the procedure.

Begin

Begin your exercise in your warm, cozy, and familiar place. Wear loose-fitting clothing and settle comfortably in your favorite chair or sofa. Always start your exercise by listening to the conversation. Remember that your heart and your brain are connected and in constant communication. Listen to your heart.

Take a deep breath in through your nose and let it out through your mouth. Count s-l-o-w-l-y to seven. Notice that when you take in a deep breath, your heart rate slightly increases, and as you exhale, your heart rate decreases. Take a few more breaths and notice this trend: in, your heart rate increases; out, your heart rate decreases. The more you practice, the better you will get at hearing your heartbeat. This is excellent proof that you are participating in the conversation.

As you begin, focus on your heart and clear your mind of any other thoughts. Liken this exercise to working out different muscles in the gym. Instead of working your back, your shoulders, or your biceps, look at this exercise as exercising and developing your heart-brain connection.

Relax

Remember that the relaxation response is a state of deep relaxation that is the opposite of the fight-or-flight response. You can reach this state by deep breathing. It is comfortable, soothing, and nurturing for your heart. Breathing in and out causes changes in the heart rate. When you take a deep breath in, you are activating the sympathetic nervous system, which causes your heart rate to speed up. When you exhale, count to seven, like the number of letters in B-R-E-A-T-H-E. This extended exhalation activates the parasympathetic nervous system and slows the heart rate by sending signals from your brain to your heart on a highway called the vagus nerve. This fluctuation or variability of the heart rate is good for the heart.

Envision

As you come to the end of a familiar path, you realize you are not alone. The entire surgical team—the operating room nurses, the surgical technologists, and the physicians—is walking on the path with you. You notice that like you, these people are familiar with the environment just as they are familiar with the operating room. Everything is calm, comfortable, and peaceful.

At the foot of a majestic river, you are joined by your surgical team, and you all take a comfortable seat. You notice that a storm has just passed and that the clouds are beginning to clear. You watch as the sun peaks through the gray clouds and reflects off the river, which after the storm is powerful and deep. As you look across the river, you notice a large oak tree, which has two large broken branches. You imagine that this damage was caused by the powerful winds of the storm, and you liken the damage to the illness for which you are having surgery.

As you look closer, notice new growth sprouting from the broken tree branches. Marvel at the reparative ability of the tree and imagine that this is similar to successfully healing from your surgery. Appreciate that the flow of the river provides the water and nutrients to the surrounding lush vegetation, and liken it to your heart supplying your tissues with oxygen. Observe that the trees are lined up together and that the gentle breeze causes them to sway synchronously and rhythmically.

Imagine how this synchronous rhythm is like your heart parts, with all the valves, arteries, and chambers working harmoniously together as an efficient pump propelling blood to all the tissues. Notice the warm sun on your shoulders and how it improves your circulation and blood flow. Imagine that the flow of the river is constant and maintained by the strength and force of the waterfall. Notice how the water level and the depth of the river are maintained and constant, like your heart in perfect balance.

Apply

Make a mental connection and apply how the sprouting branches are like your healing body. Your immune system is strong and powerful like the river. Imagine how the restorative power of nature and the return to order after the storm are similar to your body's healthy immune system, which will help you successfully heal from surgery. Note how the beautiful vegetation around you represents your healthy heart. Listen to the sounds around you: the gentle breeze blowing in the trees, the chirping of the birds, and the sound of the distant waterfall resemble your heart—constant, rhythmic, and powerful.

Treat

View this exercise as a special treatment for yourself. You are deserving of this pleasurable and therapeutic time. The exercise is pleasurable, relaxing, and rejuvenating. This is not a chore or a task. Before long you will look forward to this work and feel like a runner who experiences a high from running.

Remember that this exercise, when performed correctly, is therapeutic and serves to decrease your heart rate, lower your blood pressure, and lower your vascular tone. The deeper and more relaxed you become, the more protective and effective is the therapy. Meditation and exercises such as B-R-E-A-T-H-E technique are therapeutic: they lower the levels of cardio-toxic hormones such as cortisol and adrenaline. This exercise increases heart-rate variability and low fluctuations in heart rate (low heart-rate variability) in patients who have been diagnosed with poor cardiovascular outcomes. Recall that guided imagery bolsters the immune system, lowers blood pressure and heart rate, and decreases anxiety.

Heal

When using the B-R-E-A-T-H-E technique, imagine the healing properties of relaxation. Your deep breathing helps you to train the nerves that connect the brain and the heart and has a calming and slowing effect on your heart rate. This exercise will reduce stress and make you feel better, which will enhance healing in your body. It will allow you to downshift so that your engine can cool and idle for a while. Imagine that the warm sun on your shoulders causes your blood vessels to dilate, further improving flow and thus healing your electrical system. Store the heart-healing metaphors in your memory so they can be quickly retrieved to help protect and heal your heart in a stressful situation.

End

As you end your B-R-E-A-T-H-E exercise, recall all of the heart-healing metaphors and summarize their significance and their relationship to your healing heart. Remember the perfectly flow-ing river, the beautiful swaying trees, and the powerful water-fall. Recall the powerful river as it gently sweeps the tree to the shore. As you end your exercise, you will become aware of your surroundings and feel energized. Your heart is strong, rhythmic, and unobstructed like the river.

Final Word

B-R-E-A-T-H-E is a simple, easy-to-remember, and effective relaxation technique that can help anyone to manage stress. In addition to having many health benefits, it helps you to focus, concentrate, and organize your life. The acronym itself is a reminder of the conversation between the heart and the brain and that the key to participating is through conscious breathing.

By now you should be convinced that stress is really harmful to your overall health. With our fast-paced global world filled with daily challenges and frustrations, stress is here to stay, and it's likely to become even more prevalent.

Thus, here is what I tell my patients:

- Know your triggers.
- Listen to the conversation.
- Practice B-R-E-A-T-H-E.
- Focus: use the part of your brain developed in B-R-E-A-T-H-E.
- Choose to respond to stress productively.
- Stay in the present.
- Be grateful: love your family, your friends, and your support groups.

These simple tips will help you to weather any storm, real or emotional.

Throughout this book you've journeyed down a beautiful trail and have, I hope, enjoyed all the familiar sights and sounds on the edge of the majestic river. As the book draws to an end, you may anticipate the river ending as well.

To your surprise, however, you hear a familiar roar of the waterfall just ahead in the distance, and you realize that you're approaching another waterfall that generates tremendous flow and gives way to yet another river.

Just like your closed circulatory system, which includes your heart, your lungs, and your arteries and veins, the surrounding mountains create streams, creeks, and rivulets that continuously collect and form new waterfalls, new rivers, and new paths. So the river is continuous and never really ends.

Like life, the river changes with the seasons; sometimes it's cold and deep, and sometimes it's warm and shallow, yet it's always present, always flowing. The river is continuous and occasionally full of unexpected turns and turbulent rapids, which, like stress in our lives, we can learn to navigate. We learn that we can overcome any challenge or rapid large or small and that we are always capable of finding our way toward stiller, calmer waters. The key is to follow the current. Expect the rapids, but know that with the B-R-E-A-T-H-E technique, you will always find your way to calmer waters.

Once you've mastered the technique, teach your children, your work colleagues, your family members, your friends, your teammates, and even your foes. It will help to heal many hearts. The following quote from Ralph Waldo Emerson captures this idea fairly succinctly:

To laugh often and much;

To win the respect of intelligent people and the affection of children;

To earn the appreciation of honest critics and endure the betrayal of false friends;

To appreciate beauty, to find the best in others;

To leave the world a bit better, whether by a healthy child, a garden patch, or a redeemed social condition;

To know even one life (including yourself) has breathed easier because you have lived. This is to have succeeded.

Sources

Alexander, C. N., Robinson, P., Orme-Johnson, D. W., Schneider, R. H., and Walton, K. G. Effects of *transcendental meditation* compared to other methods of relaxation and meditation in reducing risk factors, morbidity, and mortality. *Homeostasis* 35 (1994): 243–264.

Benson, H. Systemic hypertension and the relaxation response. *New England Journal of Medicine* 296 (1977): 1152–1156.

Berenson G. S., Wattigney, W. A., Tracy R. E., et al. Atherosclerosis of the aorta and coronary arteries and cardiovascular risk factors in persons aged 6 to 30 years and studied at necropsy. (Bogalusa Heart Study). *American Journal of Cardiology* 70 (1992): 851– 858.

Birnbaum, Y., Kloner, R. A., Perritt R., et al. Atherosclerotic cardiovascular mortality during the 1992 riots in Los Angeles. *American Journal of Cardiology* 79 (1997): 1155–1158.

Blumenthal J. A., et al. Effects of exercise and stress management training on markers of cardiovascular risk in patients with ischemic heart disease, a randomized controlled trial. *Journal of the American Medical Association* 293 (2005): 1626–1634.

Boyle, S. H., et al. Hostility as a predictor of survival in patients with coronary artery disease. *Psychosomatic Medicine* 66, no. 5 (Sept. 1, 2004): 629–632.

Burg, M. M., et al. ICD shocks and emotional stress, psychological traits and emotion-triggering of ICD shock-terminated arrhythmias. *Psychosomatic Medicine* 66 (2004): 898–902.

Carlson, L. A., et al. Plasma lipids and urinary excretion of catecholamines in man during experimentally induced emotional stress, and their modification by nicotinic acid. *Journal of Clinical Investigation* 47, no. 8 (Aug. 1968): 1795–1805.

Carney, R. M., et al. Low heart rate variability and the effect of depression on post-myocardial infarction mortality. *Archives of Internal Medicine* 165 (July 11, 2005):1486–1491.

Chambers, W. N., and Reiser, M. F. Emotional stress in the precipitation of congestive heart failure. *Psychosomatic Medicine* 15 (1953): 38–60.

Chandola, T., et al. Work stress and coronary heart disease: What are the mechanisms? *European Heart Journal* 29, no. 5 (2008): 640–648.

Chesney, M. A., Agras, S., Benson, H., Blumenthal, J. A., Engel, B. T., Foreyt, J. P., Kaufmann, P. G., Levenson, R. M., Pickering, T. G., Randall, W. C., and Schwartz, P. J. Task Force 5: Nonpharmocologic approaches to the treatment of hypertension. *Circulation* 76, no. 1 (1987): 104–109.

Chi, J. S., Poole, W. K., Kandefer, S. C., et al. Cardiovascular mortality in New York City after September 11, 2001. *American Journal of Cardiology* 92 (2003): 857–861.

Christakis, N. A., and Allison, P. D. Mortality after the hospitalization of a spouse. *New England Journal of Medicine 354*, no. 7 (Feb. 16, 2006): 719–730.

Cohen S., et al. Psychological stress and susceptibility to the common cold. *New England Journal of Medicine 325*, no. 9 (Aug. 29, 1991): 606–612.

Cowan, M. J., Pike, K. C., and Budzynski, H. K. Psychosocial nursing therapy following sudden cardiac arrest: Impact on two-year survival. *Nursing Research* 50 (Mar.-Apr. 2001): 68–76.

Critchley H. D., et al. Mental stress and sudden cardiac death: Asymmetric midbrain activity as a linking mechanism. *Brain 128*, no. 1 (2005): 75–85.

Culi, V., Eterovi, D., and Miri, D. Meta-analysis of possible external triggers of acute myocardial infarction. *International Journal of Cardiology* 99 (2005): 1–8.

Danner, M., Kasl, S. V., Abramson, J. L., and Vaccarino, V. Association between depression and elevated C-reactive protein. *Psychosomatic Medicine* 66: 684–691 (2004).

Del Pozo, J. M., et al. Biofeedback treatment increases heart rate variability in patients with known coronary artery disease. *American Heart Journal* 147, no. 3 (Mar. 2004): E11.

De Vogli, R., Chandola, T., and Marmot, M. G. Negative aspects of close relationships and heart disease. *Archives of Internal Medicine* 167 (2007): 1951–1957.

Dimsdale, J. E. Psychological stress and cardiovascular disease. *Journal of the American College of Cardiology,* 51: 1237–1246 (Dec. 2007).

Dixhoorn, J. van, and White, A. Relaxation therapy for rehabilitation and prevention in ischaemic heart disease: A systematic review and meta-analysis. *European Journal of Cardiovascular Prevention & Rehabilitation* 12, no. 3 (June 2005):193–202.

Dobbels, F. Does every cardiologist need a psychologist? Transcendental meditation more effective in reducing high blood pressure compared to other stress reduction programs, study shows. *European Heart Journal* 28 (2007): 2964–2966.

Domenico, C. et al. Arrhythmogenic right ventricular dysplasia/cardiomyopathy: Need for an international registry. *Circulation* 101 (2000): 101–106.

Eaker, E. D., et al. Anger and hostility predict the development of atrial fibrillation in men in the Framingham Offspring Study. *Circulation* 109, no. 10 (Mar. 16, 2004): 1267–1271.

Enos, W. F., Holmes, R. H., and Beyer, J. Coronary disease among United States soldiers killed in action in Korea: Preliminary report. *Journal of the American Medical Association* 152 (1953): 1090–1093.

Falk, E., Shah, P. K., and Fuster, V. Coronary plaque disruption. *Circulation* 92, no. 3 (Aug. 1, 1995): 657–671.

Ford, D. E., and Erlinger, T. P. Depression and C-reactive protein in U.S. adults: Data from the Third National Health and Nutrition Examination Survey. *Archives of Internal Medicine* 164 (2004): 1010–1014.

Frasure-Smith, N., et al. Disease depression and anxiety as predictors of 2-year cardiac events in patients with stable coronary artery disease. *Archives of General Psychiatry* 65, no. 1 (2008): 62–71.

Fuster, V. Lewis A. Conner Memorial Lecture: "Mechanisms Leading to Myocardial Infarction: Insights From Studies of Vascular Biology." *Circulation* 90, no. 4 (Oct. 1994): 2126–2146.

Gelb, B. D. Marfan syndrome and related disorders: More tightly connected than we thought. *New England Journal of Medicine* 355, no. 8 (Aug. 24, 2006): 841–844.

Gidron, N., Kupper, M., Kwaijtaal, J., Winter, and Denollet, J. Vagus–brain communication in atherosclerosis-related inflammation: A neuroimmunomodulation perspective of CAD. *Atherosclerosis* 195, no. 2 (2007): E1–E9.

Goldbourt, U., Yaari, S., and Medalie, J. H. Factors predictive of long-term coronary heart disease mortality among 10,059 male Israeli civil servants and municipal employees. *Cardiology*, 82 (1993): 100–121.

Greene, W. A., Goldstein, S., and Moss, A. J. Psychosocial aspects of sudden death: A preliminary report. *Archives of Internal Medicine* 129, no. 5 (May 1972): 725–731.

Gullette, E. C., Blumenthal, J. A., Babyak, M., Jiang, W., Waugh, R. A., Frid, D. J., O'Connor, C. M., Morris, J. J., and Krantz, D. S. Effects of mental stress on myocardial ischemia during daily life. *Journal of the American Medical Association* 277, no. 19 (May 21, 1997): 1521–1526.

Hansson, G. K. Inflammation, atherosclerosis, and coronary artery disease. *New England Journal of Medicine* 352, no. 16 (Apr. 21, 2005): 1685–1695.

Hatzaras, J., et al. Role of exertion or emotion as inciting events for acute aortic dissection. *American Journal of Cardiology* 100, no. 9 (Nov. 2007): 1470–1472.

Hartikainen, J. , et al. Predictive power of heart rate variability used as a stratifier of cardiac mortality after myocardial infarction in patients discharged with and without beta-blocker therapy. *Annals of Noninvasive Electrocardiology* 1, no. 1 (Oct. 27, 2006): 12–18.

Holman, E. A., et al. Terrorism, acute stress, and cardiovascular health: A 3-year national study following the September 11th attacks. *Archives of General Psychiatry* 65, no. 1 (2008): 73–80.

Kabat-Zinn, J., Lipworth, L., and Burney, R. The clinical use of mindfulness meditation for the self-regulation of chronic pain. *Journal of Behavioral Medicine*, 8 (1985): 163–190.

Kalisch, R., et al. Neural correlates of self-distraction from anxiety and a process model of cognitive emotion regulation. *Journal of Cognitive Neuroscience* 18 (2006): 1266–1276.

Kaushik, R., Kaushik, R., Mahajan, S., and Rajesh, V. Effects of mental relaxation and slow breathing in essential hypertension. *Complementary Therapies in Medicine* 14, no 2 (2006): 120–126.

Kawachi, I., Colditz, G. A., Ascherio, A., et al. Prospective study of phobic anxiety and risk of coronary heart disease in men. *Circulation* 89 (1994): 1992–1997.

Klaus, L., Beniaminovitz, A., Choi, L., Greenfield, F., Whitworth, G. C., Oz, M. C., and Mancini, D. M. Pilot study of guided imagery use in patients with severe heart failure. *American Journal of Cardiology* 86, no. 1 (July 1, 2000): 101–104.

Kloner, R. A. The "Merry Christmas Coronary" and "Happy New Year Heart Attack" phenomenon. *Circulation* 110, no. 25 (Dec. 21, 2004): 3744–3745.

———. Natural and unnatural triggers of myocardial infarction. *Progressive Cardiovascular Disease* 48 (2006): 285–300.

Kloner, R. A., Poole W. K., Perritt R. L., et al. When throughout the year is coronary death most likely to occur? A 12-year population-based analysis of more than 222,000 cases. *Circulation* 100 (1999): 1630–1634.

Kop, W. J. Chronic and acute psychological risk factors for clinical manifestations of coronary artery disease. *Psychosomatic Medicine* 61, no. 4 (July 1, 1999): 476–487.

Kshettry, V. R., Carole, L. F., Henly, S. J., et al. Complementary alternative medical therapies for heart surgery patients: Feasibility, safety, and impact. *Annals of Thoracic Surgery* 81, no. 1 (Jan. 2006): 201–205.

Kubzansky, L. D., Kawachi, I., Spiro, A., et al. Is worrying bad for your heart? A prospective study of worry and coronary heart disease in the Normative Aging Study. *Circulation* 95 (1997): 818–824.

Kubzansky, L. D., Kawachi, I., Weiss, S. T., and Sparrow, D. Anxiety and coronary heart disease: A synthesis of epidemiological, psychological, and experimental evidence. *Annals of Behavioral Medicine* 20 (1998): 47–58.

Kubzansky, L. D., et al. Emotional vitality and incident coronary heart disease: Benefits of healthy psychological functioning. *Archives of General Psychiatry* 64, no. 12 (Dec. 2007): 1393–401.

Lewis, A. Mechanisms leading to myocardial infarction: Insights from studies of vascular biology. Paper presented at the Department of Epidemiology and Public Health, University College, London.

Leor, J., Poole, W. K., Kloner, R. A., et al. Sudden cardiac death triggered by an earthquake. *New England Journal of Medicine* 334 (1996): 413–415.

Leserman, J., Stuart, E. M., Mamish, M. E., and Benson, H. The efficacy of the relaxation response in preparing for cardiac surgery. *Behavioral Medicine* 5 (Fall 1989): 111–117.

Levine, S. P., et al. Platelet activation and secretion associated with emotional stress. *Circulation* 71 (1985): 1129–1134.

Linden, W., Phillips, M. J., and Leclerc, J. Psychological treatment of cardiac patients: A meta-analysis. Paper presented at the University of Regina, Saskatchewan, Canada, Nov. 2007.

Maron, B. J. Sudden death in young athletes: Lessons from the Hank Gathers affair. *New England Journal of Medicine* 329 (1993): 55–77.

Maron, B. J., Shirani, J., Poliac, L. C., Mathenge, R., Roberts, W. C., and Mueller, F. O. Sudden death in young competitive athletes: Clinical, demographic, and pathologic profiles. *Journal of the American Medical Association* 276 (1996): 199–204.

Matthews, K. A., Gump, B. B., Harris, K. F., Haney, T. L., and Barefoot, J. C. Hostile behaviors predict cardiovascular mortality among men enrolled in the Multiple Risk Factor Intervention Trial. *Circulation* 109 (2004): 66–70.

McGill, H.C., et al. Origin of atherosclerosis in childhood and adolescence. *American Journal of Clinical Nutrition* 72, no. 5, (November 2000): 1307S–1315s.

McNamara, J. J., Molot, M. A., Stremple, J. F., and Cutting, R. T. Coronary artery disease in combat casualties in Vietnam. *Journal of the American Medical Association* 216 (1971): 1185–1187.

Meisel, S. R., Kutz, I., Dayan, K. I., et al. Effect of Iraqi missile war on incidence of acute myocardial infarction and sudden death in Israeli civilians. *Lancet* 338 (1991): 660–661.

Melamed, S. Life stress, emotional reactivity, and their relation to plasma lipids in employed women. *Evidence-Based Mental Health* 4 (2001): 108

Middlekauff, H. R., et al. Impact of acute mental stress on sympathetic nerve activity and regional blood flow in advanced heart failure: Implications for triggering adverse cardiac events. *Circulation* 96, no. 6 (Sept. 16, 1997): 1835–1842.

Mittleman, M. A., et al. Triggering of acute myocardial infarction onset by episodes of anger. *Circulation* 92, no. 7 (Oct. 1, 1995): 1720–1725.

Muller, J. E., Abela, G. S., Nesto, R. W., et al. Triggers, acute factors, and vulnerable plaques: The lexicon of a new frontier. *Journal of the American College of Cardiology* 23 (1994): 809–813.

Myeong Soo Lee, Mo Kyung Kim, and LeeYong-Heum. Effects of QI-therapy (External Qigong) on cardiac autonomic tone: A randomized placebo controlled study. *International Journal of Neuroscience* 115, no. 9 (2005): 1345–1350.

Nimchinsky, E. A., et al. A neuronal morphologic type unique to humans and great apes. *Proceedings of the National Academy of Sciences* 96, no. 9 (Apr. 27, 1999): 5268–5273.

Ornish, D., et al. Intensive lifestyle changes for reversal of coronary heart disease. *Journal of the American Medical Association* 280 (1998): 2001–2007.

Orth-Gomer, K., Wamala, S. P., Horsten, M., Schenck-Gustafsson, K., Shneiderman, N., and Mittleman, M. A. Marital stress worsens prognosis in women with coronary heart disease: The Stockholm Female Coronary Risk Study. *Journal of the American Medical Association* 284, no. 23 (Dec. 20, 2000): 3008–3014.

Palinkas, L. A. Psychosocial therapy (relaxation therapy) reduced the risk of cardiovascular death at 2 years after "out of hospital" sudden cardiac arrest. *Evidence-Based Mental Health* 4(2001): 108.

Palinski, W., and Napoli, C. The fetal origins of atherosclerosis: Maternal hypercholesterolemia and cholesterol-lowering or antioxidant treatment during pregnancy influence in utero programming and postnatal susceptibility to atherogenesis. *FASEB Journal* 16 (2002): 1348–1360.

Pedersen, S. S., et al. Type D personality is associated with increased anxiety and depressive symptoms in patients with an implantable cardioverter defibrillator and their partners. *Psychosomatic Medicine* 66, no. 5 (Sept. 1, 2004): 714–719.

Pignalberi, C., Ricci, R., and Santini, M. Psychological stress and sudden death. *Italian Heart Journal Supplement* 3, no. 10 (Oct. 2002): 1011–1021.

Poole, W. K., Chi, J. S., Walton, J. D., et al. Increased cardiovascular mortality associated with the turn of the millennium in Los Angeles County, California. *Journal of Epidemiological Community Health* 59 (2005): 205–206.

Puli, V., Eterovi, D., Miri, D., Giunio, L., Lukin, A., and Fabijani, D. Triggering of ventricular tachycardia by meteorologic and emotional stress: Protective effect of {beta}-blockers and anxiolytics in men and elderly. *American Journal of Epidemiology* 160, no. 11 (Dec. 1, 2004): 1047–1058.

Rosenstock, L., et al. Firefighting and death from cardiovascular causes. *New England Journal of Medicine* 356, no. 12 (Mar. 22, 2007): 1261–1263.

Rozanski, A., Bairey, C. N, Krantz, D. S., Friedman, J., Resser, K. J., Morell, M., Hilton-Chalfen, S., Hestrin, L., Bietendorf, J., and Berman, D. S. Mental stress and the induction of silent myocardial ischemia in patients with coronary artery disease. *New England Journal of Medicine* 318, no. 16 (Apr. 21, 1988): 1005–1012.

Rugulies, R. Depression as a predictor for coronary heart disease: A review and meta-analysis. *American Journal of Preventive Medicine* 23 (2002): 51–61.

Selzer, A., and Cohn, K. E. Natural history of mitral stenosis: A review. *Circulation* 45 (1972): 878–890.

Shedd, O. L., et al. The World Trade Center attack: Increased frequency of defibrillator shocks for ventricular arrhythmias in patients living remotely from New York City. *Journal of the American College of Cardiology* 44, no. 6 (Sept. 15, 2004): 1265–1267.

Shen, B. J., et al. Anxiety characteristics independently and prospectively predict myocardial infarction. *Journal of the American College of Cardiology* 51 (2008): 113–115.

Smoller, J. W., et al. Panic attacks and risk of incident cardiovascular events among postmenopausal women in the Women's Health Initiative Observational Study. *Archives of General Psychiatry* 64, no. 10 (2007): 1153–1160.

Sternberg, E. M. *Walter B. Cannon and* "Voodoo' Death": A perspective from 60 years on. *American Journal of Public Health* 92, no. 10 (Oct. 2002): 1564–1566.

Strike, P. C., Perkins-Porras, L., Whitehead, D. L., et al. Triggering of acute coronary syndromes by physical exertion and anger: Clinical and sociodemographic characteristics. *Heart* 92 (2006): 1035–1040.

Strike, P. C., and Steptoe, A. Behavioral and emotional triggers of acute coronary syndromes: A systematic review and critique. *Psychosomatic Medicine* 67 (2005): 179–186.

Strong, J. P., Malcom, G. T., McMahan, C. A., Tracy, R. E., Newman, W. P., Herdeick, E. E., and Cornhill, J. F. Prevalence and extent of atherosclerosis in adolescents and young adults: Implications for prevention from the pathobiological determinants of atherosclerosis in youth study. *Journal of the American Medical Association* 281 (1999): 727–735.

Sudsuang, R., Chentanez, V., and Veluvan, K. Effect of Buddhist meditation on serum cortisol and total protein levels, blood pressure, pulse rate, lung volume and reaction time. *Physiology & Behavior,* 50 (1991): 543–548.

Suls, J., and Bunde, J. Anger, anxiety, and depression as risk factors for cardiovascular disease: The problems and implications of overlapping affective dispositions. *Psychological Bulletin* 131 (2005): 260–300.

Taylor, C. B., Farquhar, J. W., Nelson, E., and Agras, S. Relaxation therapy and high blood pressure. *Archives of General Psychiatry* 34 (1977): 339–342.

Thaddeus, W., et al. Increased stress-induced inflammatory responses in male patients with major depression and increased early life stress. *Archives of General Psychiatry* 65 (2008): 409–415.

Thiene, G., Nava, A., Corrado, D., Rossi, L., and Pennelli, N. Right ventricular cardiomyopathy and sudden death in young people. *New England Journal of Medicine* 318 (1988): 129–133.

Todaro, J. F., Shen, B .J., Niaura, R., Spiro, A., and Ward, K. D. Effect of negative emotions on frequency of coronary heart disease.

(Normative Aging Study). *American Journal of Cardiology* 92 (2003): 901–906.

Toker, S., Shirom, A., Shapira, I., Berliner, S., and Melamed, S. M. The association between burnout, depression, anxiety, and inflammation biomarkers: C-reactive protein and fibrinogen in men and women. *Journal of Occupational Health Psychology* 2 (2005): 275–288.

Tuzcu, E. M., Kapadia, S. R., Tutar, E., et al. High prevalence of coronary atherosclerosis in asymptomatic teenagers and young adults: Evidence from intravascular ultrasound. *Circulation* 103 (2001): 2705–2715.

Viskin, S., and Belhassen, B. When you only live twice. *New England Journal of Medicine* 332, no. 18 (May 4, 1995): 1221–1225.

Wilbert-Lampen, U., et al. Cardiovascular events during World Cup soccer. *New England Journal of Medicine* 358, no. 5 (Jan. 31, 2008): 475–483.

Williams, J. E., Paton, C. C., Siegler, I. C., Eigenbrodt, M. L., Nieto, F. J., and Tyroler, H. A. Anger proneness predicts coronary heart disease risk: Prospective analysis from the Atherosclerosis Risk In Communities (ARIC) Study. *Circulation* 101, no. 17 (May 2, 2000): 2034–2039.

Witte, D. R., Bots, M. L., Hoes, A. W., and Grobbee, D. E. Cardiovascular mortality in Dutch men during 1996 European football championship: Longitudinal population study. *British Medical Journal* 321, no. 7276 (Dec. 23, 2000): 1552–1554.

Wittstein, I. S., et al. Neurohumoral features of myocardial stunning due to sudden emotional stress. *New England Journal of Medicine* 352, no. 6 (Feb. 10, 2005): 539–548.

Wulsin, L. R., and Singal, B. M. Do depressive symptoms increase the risk for the onset of coronary disease? A systematic quantitative review. *Psychosomatic Medicine* 65 (2003): 201–210.

Yarnell, J. Stress at work: An independent risk factor for coronary heart disease? *European Heart Journal* 29 (2008): 579–580.

Yusuf, S., et al. Effect of potentially modifiable risk factors associated with myocardial infarction in 52 countries (the INTERHEART study): Case-control study. *Lancet* 364, no. 9438 (Sept. 11, 2004): 937–952.

Zamarra, J. W., Schneider, R. H., Besseghini, I., Robinson, D. K., and Salerno, J. W. Usefulness of the transcendental meditation program in the treatment of patients with coronary artery disease. *American Journal of Cardiology* 77, no. 10 (Apr. 15, 1996): 867–870.

Ziegelstein, R. C. Acute emotional stress and cardiac arrhythmias. *Journal of the American Medical Association* 298, no. 3 (2007): 324–329.

Ziegelstein, R. C. Acute emotional stress and the heart. *Journal of the American Medical Association* 298 (2007): 360.

Zieske, A. W., Malcom, G. T., and Strong, J. P. Natural history and risk factors of atherosclerosis in children and youth: The PDAY study. *Pediatric Pathology and Molecular Medicine* 21 (2002): 213–237.

Zimetbaum, P., et al. Evaluation of patients with palpitations. *New England Journal of Medicine* 338, no. 19 (May 7, 1998): 1369–1373.

Suggested Reading

Achterberg, Jeanne. *Rituals of Healing: Using Imagery for Health and Wellness.* New York: Bantam Books, 1994.

Begley, Sharon. *Train Your Mind, Change Your Brain.* New York: Ballantine Books, 2007.

Benson, Herbert. *The Relaxation Response.* New York: Harper Torch, 1976.

Childre, Doc. *Transforming Anxiety.* Oakland, CA: New Harbinger, 2006.

Goleman, Daniel. *Emotional Intelligence: Why It Can Matter More Than IQ.* New York: Bantam Dell, 1994.

———. *Social Intelligence: The New Science of Human Relationships.* New York: Bantam Dell, 2006.

Gupta, Sanjay. *Chasing Life.* New York: Warner Wellness, 2007.

Gurneri, Mimi. *The Heart Speaks.* New York: Touchstone, 2006.

Kabat-Zinn, Jon. *Full Catastrophe Living: Using the Wisdom of Your Body and Mind to Face Stress, Pain, and Illness.* New York: Bantam Dell, 1990.

Ornish, Dean. *The Spectrum: A Scientifically Proven Program to Feel Better, Live Longer, Lose Weight, and Gain Health.* New York: Ballantine Books, 2007.

Oz, Mehmet. *Healing from the Heart.* New York: Plume, 1999.

Rossman, Martin. *Guided Imagery for Self Healing*. Tiburon, CA: HJ Kramer, 2000.

Sapolsky, Robert. *Why Zebras Don't Get Ulcers*. New York: Owl Books, 1994.

Weil, Andrew. *Healthy Aging: A Lifelong Guide to Your Well-Being*. New York: Anchor Books, 2005.

Index

Printed in the USA
CPSIA information can be obtained
at www.ICGtesting.com
JSHW012024140824
68134JS00033B/2859